J. Chrubasik M. Cousins E. Martin (Eds.)

Advances in Pain Therapy I

Springer-Verlag
Berlin Heidelberg New York
London Paris Tokyo
Hongkong Barcelona
Budapest

J. Chrubasik, M. D.
E. Martin, M. D.
Department of Anesthesiology
University of Heidelberg
Im Neuenheimer Feld 110
D-6900 Heidelberg, FRG

M. Cousins, M. D.
Professor of Anaesthesia
Dept. of Anesthesiology
University Hospital Sydney
Sydney, Australia

ISBN-13: 978-3-540-55536-0 **e-ISBN-13: 978-3-642-77555-0**
DOI: 10.1007/978-3-642-77555-0

Printed and Binding: Druckhaus Beltz, 6944 Hemsbach
27/3145/5 4 3 2 1 0 – Printed on acid-free paper

Contents

List of Contributors

Prof. Dr. D. Carr
Dept. of Anesthesiology, Harvard Medical School,
Boston, USA

Prof. Dr. J. Chrubasik
Dept. of Anesthesiology, University Hospital,
Heidelberg, Germany

Dr. S. Chrubasik
Dept. of Forensic Medicine, University Hospital,
Freiburg, Germany

Prof. Dr. M. Cousins
Dept. of Anesthesiology, University of Sydney,
Sydney, Australia

Dr. U. Dethlefsen
Institute of Clinical Research,
Hamburg, Germany

Prof. Dr. M. Lazorthes
Dept. of Neurosurgery, University Hospital,
Toulouse, France

Prof. Dr. E. Martin
Dept. of Anesthesiology, University Hospital,
Heidelberg, Germany

Dr. D. Niv
Dept. of Anesthesiology, Ichilov Hospital,
Tel Aviv, Israel

Prof. Dr. W. Parris
Dept. of Anesthesiology, Vanderbilt University,
Nashville, USA

Prof. Dr. R. Penn
Dept. of Neurosurgery, University Hospital,
Chicago, USA

Prof. Dr. P. Rosenberg
Dept. of Anesthesiology, University Hospital,
Helsinki, Finland

Preface

E. Martin

Since chronic pain therapy was introduced by J. Bonica in 1961, efforts have been made world-wide to establish basic concepts for the treatment of chronic malignancy- or non-malignancy-related pain. Thirty years later many patients continue to suffer from intractable back pain, headache, facial and postherpetic neuralgia, central poststroke pain, fibromyalgia, pain resulting from terminal illness, and pain inadequately relieved despite the availability of effective treatments that would afford these patients an improved quality of life. The lack of specialists familiar with recent devlopments contributes to the number of patients with "refractory" pain. World-wide, there is a sustained demand for interdisciplinary pain clinics and a need for special training programs.

Careful history-taking and analysis of the pain are the key to successful treatment and avoid the subjection of patients to unsuccessful therapies. Basic knowledge of the clinical pharmacology of analgesics, both opioid and nonopioid, is essential, and the WHO directives on drug administration provide important official guidelines. Only when basic principles are adhered to can effective analgesic treatment be provided. New formulae for slow analgesic release, such as MST continous, alleviate the stress of out-patient treatment and increase the patient's independence. Other techniques such as the epidural, intrathecal, or intraventricular modes of administration, dorsal column stimulation, radiofrequency for dorsal root ganglia lesions, and the intrapleural technique are alternative methods for the management of intractable pain and require special skills. Education of doctors and nurses is therefore fundamental to providing satisfactory pain relief.

Evaluation of transcutaneous electrical nerve stimulation and acupuncture is difficult and the efficacy of these methods has yet to be established. Controlled trials are required to investigate the role of spinal peptides for treatment of pain. Pain management programs should also include behavioral therapy to alleviate psychosomatic pain. The main areas of pain clinic activity are in the field of pain physiology, neuropharmacology, and psychology. The papers collected in this book provide an update on the various methods in pain management and should serve as a useful guide for training programs.

The Pain Clinic and Cancer Pain Treatment

MICHAEL J. COUSINS

Cancer Pain and the Pain Clinic Specialist

The treatment of cancer pain has gained worldwide impetus, partly as a result of dedicated individuals in pain clinics who have an interest in cancer pain treatment, but more significantly as a result of more generalised initiatives. In 1984 the World Health Organisation (WHO) denoted cancer pain as a major world health problem and in 1989 the International Association for the Study of Pain (IASP) formed an official relationship with the WHO to mount a global programme to improve the treatment of cancer pain [3]. Since the pioneering work of Dame Cicely Saunders in the UK and Balfour Mount in Canada, palliative medicine has gradually grown in strength to the point where the first comprehensive text on this subject will be published in 1992 [5]. Specialist oncology bodies in some countries have now substantially increased the emphasis on cancer pain treatment in the training of oncologists in their speciality examinations, and in the USA assessment of pain is mandatory in cancer research projects funded by the National Cancer Institute.

A very positive aspect of all of the foregoing developments is that many more patients are now receiving effective treatment of their cancer pain. Also, there has been a much more vigorous approach to the wider aspects of palliative medicine, of which pain control is only a part. As a result, some oncologists and palliative care physicians feel that pain control can only be effectively addressed in the context of all of the other symptoms experienced by patients with cancer. In some centres this has led to a reluctance to refer any patients with cancer pain to a pain clinic. This is by no means a theoretical problem, since it has resulted in a dramatic change in the scope of activity for some pain clinics which previously contributed substantially to the treatment of cancer pain. This many have been an initial over-reaction; however, it will continue in some form since the patients are under the control of oncologists who liaise very closely with palliative care physicians. The challenge for pain clinics is to identify those patients who can be particularly helped by the range of personnel and expertise available in individual pain clinic settings. Many anaesthesiologists have learnt that this can only be achieved by very close liaison with oncologists, by attending

Table 1. Pain syndromes in patients with cancer: pain directly caused by cancer (primary or metastatic). (From [1])

Mechanism	Common sites and characteristics of pain
Infiltration of bone by tumor	Dull, constant aching ± muscle spasm
Base of skul (jugular foramen, clivus, sphenoid sinus)	Early onset pain in occiput, vertex, frontal areas, respectively
Vertebral body (subluxation atlas, metastases C7–T1, L1 sacral)	Early onset pain in neck and skull, neck and shoulders, midback, lower back, and coccyx, respectively ± neurologica deficit
Metastatic fracture close to nerves	Acute onset pain + muscle spasm
Infiltration or compression of nerve tissue by tumor	
Peripheral nerve (± peripheral and perivascular lymphangitis)	Burning constant pain in area of peripheral sensory loss ± dysesthesia and hyperalgesia ± signs of sympathetic over-activity. See neuropathy definition
Plexus, *e.g.*, lumbar	Radicular pain to anterior thigh and groin (L1–L3) or to leg and foot (L4–S2)
e.g., sacral	Dull aching midline perianal pain + sacral sensory loss and fecal and urinary incontinence.
e.g., brachial	Radicular pain in shoulder and arm ± Homer's syndrome (superior pulmonary sulcus or Pancoast syndrome)
Meningeal carcinomatosis	Constant headache ± neck stiffness or low back and buttock pain
Epidural spinal cord compression (± vertebral body infiltration)	Severe neck and back pain locally over involved vertebra, or radicular pain
Obstruction of hollow viscus *e.g.*, gut, genitourinary tract)	Poorly localized, dull, sickening pain, typical visceral pain
Occlusion of arteries and veins by tumor	Ischemic pain like rest pain (skin) or claudication (muscle) or pain ± venous engorgement
Stretching of periosteum or fascia, in tissues with tight investment, ba tumefaction	Severe localized pain *(e.g., periosteum)* or typical visceral pain *(e.g., ovary)*
Inflammation owing to necrosis and infection of tumors (± superficial ulceration)	Severe localized pain *(e.g., perineum)*, visceral pain *(e.g., cervix)*
Soft tissue infiltration	Localized pain; unsightly and foul-smelling if ulcerated
Raised intracranial pressure	Severe constant headache, behavioral changes, confusion, etc.

* A subcategory can be defined as "Pain related to the cancer", e.g., muscle spasm, constipation, bedsores, lymphedema, candidiasis, herpetic and postherpetic neuralgia, deep venous thrombosis, pulmonary embolism.

appropriate oncology rounds and, if possible, by developing a formal relationship with palliative care and oncology units.

In the view of this author, there stands to gain much by the cancer patient having access, when needed, to a multidisciplinary pain management unit.

Table 2. Pain syndromes in patients with cancer: pain associated with cancer therapy. (From [1])

Mechanism	Common sites and characteristics of pain
Following surgery	
Acute postoperative pain	Wound or referred pain; back or other sites (owing to posture during surgery)
Nerve trauma	Neuralgic pain in area of peripheral nerve or spinal nerve
Entrapment of nerves in scar tissue	Superficial wound scar, hypersensitivity of area supplied by scarred nerves (*e.g.*, perineum)
Amputation of limb or other area (*e.g.*, breast)	Localized stump pain (neuroma) or phantom pain referred to absent region
Following radiotherapy	
Acute lesions or inflammation of nerves or plexuses	Pain associated with motor and sensory loss
Radiation fibrosis of nerves or plexuses	*e.g.*, brachial plexus, lumbar plexus distribution; diffuse limb pain, 6 months to many years after radiation ± lymphedema and local skin changes ± sensory loss ± motor loss (difficult to distinguish from tumor recurrence)
Myelopathy of spinal cord	Brown-Séquard syndrome (ipsilateral sensory and contralateral motor loss) with pain at level of spinal cord damage or referred pain
Peripheral nerve tumors owing to radiation	Painful enlarging mass in area of radiation along line of peripheral nerve or plexus
Following chemotherapie	
Vinca alkaloid (vincinstine > vinblasine)-induced peripheral neuropathy	Burning pain in hands and feet associated with symmetrical polyneuropathy
Steroid pseudorheumatism owing to slow as well as rapid withdrawal of steroid treatment	Diffuse joint and muscle pain with associated tenderness to palpation but no inflammatory signs Pain resolves when steroid reinstituted.
Aseptic necrosis of bone (femoral or humoral head) with chronic steroid therapy	Pain in knee, leg, or shoulder with limitation of movement; bone scan changes delayed after pain onset
Postherpetic neuralgia, following herpes zoster infection in areal of tumor or area of radiotherapy with onset during chemotherapy	Continuous burning pain in area of sensory loss *or* Painful dysesthesias *or* Intermittent, shocklike pain

Patients with cancer do develop a wide range of chronic pain syndromes which may be either directly due to the cancer, due to cancer treatment, unrelated or indirectly related to cancer or treatment, or due to psychological factors (Tables 1–4) [1]. Sometimes such pain problems can be difficult to

Table 3. Pain syndromes in patients with cancer: pain unrelated to cancer or cancer therapy. (From [1])

Mechanism	Common sites and characteristics of pain
Neuropathy (*e.g.*, diabetic)	Burning pain in hands, feet
Degenerative disk disease	Back pain ± radicular pain
Rheumatoid arthritis	Joint pain, on movement
Diffuse osteoporosis	Back pain, limb pain (may be like causalgia)
Posture abnormalities after surgery	Back pain and muscle spasm ± radicular pain
Myofascial syndromes owing to anxiety	Local pain in muscle with muscle spasm ± referred pain; trigger areas in muscle
Headache	Typical migraine or tension type

Table 4. Pain syndromes in patients with cancer: pain exacerbated or entirely caused by psychological factors. (From [1])

Psychological factor	Possible causes
Anxiety	Sleeplessness
	Fear of death; loss of dignity (loss of self-control
	Fear of surgical mutilation; uncontrollable pain
	Fear of the future; loss of social position and work
	Confused understanding of disease owing to poor communication
	Family and financial problems
Depression	Sleeplessness
	Loss of physical abilities
	Sense of helplessness
	Disfigurement
	Loss of valued social position; financial problems
Anger	Frustration with therapeutic failures
	Resentment of sickness
	Irritability caused by pain and general discomfort

A vicious cycle usualy develops:

ANXIETY

↗ ↑ ↘

SLEEPLESSNESS ← PAIN → ANGER

↓

DEPRESSION

diagnose and resemble very much the spectrum of problems seen in chronic non-cancer pain. Here the expertise of the range of personnel available to a multidisciplinary pain management unit can be invaluable.

In cancer pain, nociceptive, neuropathic, psychological and environmental factors can all play a part, as they do in chronic non-cancer pain [8].

Some cancer specialists either fail to recognise or give too little emphasis to the possible contribution of these four important areas. Pain clinics have an important part to play in evaluating patients from this wide perspective and also in education of undergraduate and postgraduate health professionals about this broad perspective of pain [5]. The pain clinic remains the only resource where the entire focus is on pain management, education and research. It is all too apparent that there are some cancer pain problems which are still difficult or impossible to treat, and thus there remains a very important role for the pain clinic in conducting research into cancer pain and its treatment.

Facilities Required for Cancer Pain Treatment

Pain clinics have now evolved through the stage where they could operate from "multi-user" clinical space with no dedicated space of their own. To play an effective role in the treatment of cancer pain, pain clinic should provide ready access to cancer patients, preferably without requiring them to go through the usual hospital bureaucracy. THus, ideally, they should have a separate entrance at ground floor level which permits ambulances and cars easily to deposit patients and collect them. As much as possible, treatment should be provided on a "day care" basis, although preferably some dedicated inpatient beds should be available. The main ingredients of the pain clinic facilities are: an area containing standard consulting rooms; an open plan area for treatments such as nerve blocks, physiotherapy, pharmacokinetic studies for drug optimisation, teaching relaxation and other psychologic strategies, etc; offices for clinic staff, including an office for a designated clinic director; a large enough area to accommmodate the "pain conference" as well as educational activities for patients and staff; a fully equipped operating room to enable the full range of pain-relieving procedure, including unrestricted access to an image intensifier; other support rooms to allow the smooth functioning of the consulting, diagnostic and treatment procedures. Ideally this facility should be located very close to some dedicated inpatient beds for the treatment of cancer and chronic pain.

Organisation, Staffing and Educational Aspects

The IASP publication "Desirable Characteristics for Pain Treatment Facilities" sets out a sound basis for the staffing, organisation and operation of an effective pain clinic [6]. The principles outlined in this document are certainly applicable to the treatment of patients with cancer pain in a pain clinic. The ISAP guidelines recognise that resources will vary in different parts of the world, as will some aspects of practice. However, the broad principles are important, and this author believes that they are the basis of an effective contribution by the pain clinic to the treatment of cancer pain.

As is the case with some chronic pain problems, not every patient referred to a pain clinic requires the services of a large number of health care professionals; indeed a significant number of cancer pain problems can be managed by the expertise of a single individual. However, many cancer pain patients do require the services of multiple disciplines and thus the resources and range of techniques available in a pain clinic [2, 4]. In order to clarify the function and role of "pain clinics", the IASP developed the "desirable characteristics for pain treatment facilites". It is worthwhile clarifying the terms used:

1. *Pain treatment facility*. This is a generic term used to described all forms of pain treatment facilities.
2. *Multidisciplinary pain centre*. This is the most comprehensive facility, with a broad range of health care professionals and basic scientists and with activities that include research, theaching and patient care, relevant to all forms of pain, including acute pain, cancer pain and chronic non-cancer pain. Such centres are essential to the further development of pain treatment, education and research. An important aspect of such a centre is the ability to provide comprehensive assessment of the physical, psychological and environmental factors which are involved in individual patient's pain problems. Another important ingredient is an organisation which permits the members of the treatment team to communicate with each other face to face on a regular basis, both about specific patients and about overall development.
3. *Multidisciplinary pain clinic*. This differs only from a multidisciplinary pain centre in that it does not include research and teaching activities in its regular programme.
4. *Pain clinic*. The absence of interdisciplinary assessment and management distinguished this type of facility from a multidisciplinary centre or pain clinic. However, appropriate arrangements must be in place for a suitable range of consultative and therapeutic services. "Pain clinic" should never be a label for an isolated solo practitioner. However, some pain clinics may specialise in specific diagnoses or in pain related to a specific region of the body.
5. *Modality oriented clinic*. This is a facility which offers a specific type of treatment and does not provide comprehensive assessment or management. Examples would include nerve block clinics, transcutaneous nerve stimulation clinics, acupuncture clinics, and so on.

References

1. Cousins MJ (1988) Introduction to acute and chronic pain: implications for neural blockade. In: Cousins MJ, Bridenbaugh PO (eds) Neural blockade in clinical anesthesia and management of pain, 2nd ed. Lippincott, Philadelphia, pp 739–790
2. Cousins MJ (1988) Chronic pain and neurolytic neural blockade. In: Cousins MJ, Bridenbaugh PO (eds) Neural blockade in clinical anesthesia and management of pain, 2nd ed. Lippincott, Philadelphia, pp 1053–1084

3. Cousins MJ (1991) IASP Presidential address. Current status of the field of pain and of IASP in: Bond M, Charlton JE, Wollf, CJ (eds) Proceedings of the 6th world congress on pain. Elsevier, Amsterdam
4. Cousins MJ, Cherry DA, Gourlay GK (1988) Acute and chronic pain: use of spinal opioids. In: Cousins MJ, Bridenbaugh PO (eds) Neural blockade in clinical anesthesia and management of pain, 2nd ed. Lippincott, Philadelphia, pp955–1030
5. Doyle E, Hanks GW, MacDonald N (eds) (1992) Oxford Textbook of palliative medicine. Oxford University Press, Oxford
6. Lasp (1991) Core curriculum for professional education in pain. IASP, Seattle
7. IASP (1991) Desirable characteristics for pain treatment facilities and standards for physician fellowship in pain management. IASP Seattle
8. Loeser J, Cousins MD (1990) Contemporary pain management. Med J Aust 153:208–216
9. Swarm RA, Cousins MJ (1992) Anaesthetic techniques for pain control. In: Doyle E, Hanks GW, MacDonald N (eds) Oxford textbook of palliative medicine. Oxford University Press, Oxford

The WHO Concept of Cancer Pain Treatment: A Guideline Prototype and Its Context

DANIEL B. CARR

Introduction

The importance of cancer in public health is profound. This year in the United States alone, the American Cancer Society estimates there will be 520000 deaths and 1130000 new cases diagnosed [1]. In the absence of efforts directed at palliation, severe cancer pain will emerge in the majority of advanced cases [6, 9, 21]. In 1980 the WHO started a three-part program with the aim of preventing cancers with known causes, improving detection and cure rates of cancer, and relieving cancer pain [19]. The third component progressed during 1981 with the gathering of survey data in five countries (Brazil, India, Israel, Japan and Sri Lanka) that confirmed the widespread inadequacy of cancer pain relief throughout the world. In 1982 a special consultation was convened in Milan, Italy, at which the 1981 survery participants were joined by six experts on the treatment of pain and together prepared draft guidelines upon which the "Method for Cancer Pain Relief" – Annex 1 in the initial WHO document – ultimately was based. From 1981 to the publication of the first edition of *Cancer Pain Relief* in 1986, field testing and further consultation were carried out, to assure that the first edition was a carefully conceived and polished document.

Postrelease validation studies have established the effectiveness of the WHO method for cancer pain relief. Adherence to its recommendations will result in only a minority of patients with terminal cancer experiencing severe or worse pain, and most will have minimal to moderate pain [12, 16, 20, 22, 23]. Feedback from practitioners, and the need to consider ongoing therapeutic advances, dictated the preparation of a second edition that has just been released. Because this second edition has just entered the dissemination process, and bears many more similarities to than differences from the first edition, the comments below will be based upon the first edition of the WHO publication.

The purpose of this paper is to complement others in this volume by focussing on two distinct aspects of the WHO guidelines. First, it will seek to place the process of preparation of the WHO guidelines into the broader context of guideline preparation in general, and cancer pain guidelines in particular. At present, an abundance of guidelines – over 1000 in the United

States alone – have been introduced to deal with numerous issues of clinical practice, and the process of guideline development has received increasing attention as a significant one within health services and health policy research. Second, it will briefly present the key features of the WHO method for relief of cancer pain as a basis for discussion and comparison with other approaches that may be adopted in future cancer pain treatment guidelines.

The Guideline Phenomenon

Practice guidelines have recently been defined by an expert committee convened by the Institute of Medicine (IOM) of the US National Academy of Sciences as "systematically developed statements to assist practitioner and patient decisions about appropriate health care for specific clinical circumstances" [10]. "Findings and conclusions" of the same expert group included the following statement concerning the state of the art of guideline development:

"The process of systematic development, implementation, and evaluation of practice guidelines based on rigorous clinical research and soundly generated professional consensus, although progressing, has deficiencies in method, scope, and substance. Conflicts in terminology and technique characterize the field; they are notable for the confusion they create and for what they reflect about differences in values, experiences, and interests among different parties. Public and private development activities are multiplying, but the means for coordinating these efforts to resolve inconsistencies, fill in gaps, track applications and results, and assess the soundness of particular guidelines are limited. Disproportionately more attention is paid to developing guidelines than to implementing or evaluating them. Moreover, efforts to develop guidelines are necessarily constrained by inadequacies in the quality and quantity of scientific evidence on the effectiveness of many services."

As the IOM points out, guidelines for clinical practice are hardly new, as they have for millennia formed a cornerstone of organized medical education and certification. Egyptian papyri, the writings of Hippocrates, Avicenna, and Galen, and countless other manuscripts would no doubt have been considered by their authors to be "systematically developed," even though they fall short of present-day standards for evidence and documentation of the process by which clinical recommendations are distilled from clinical evidence [17]. Medical texts are also in essence guidelines.

At present, given the insistence of health insurers, managers, regulators, and consumers in reviewing care on a prospective or concurrent basis, the process of guideline development is a rapidly maturing and increasingly rigorous discipline. Guideline development is now a field of medical social science populated by economists, sociologists, political scientists and "methodologists." Medical societies have for some years been leaders in the process of guideline development. In the USA medical groups such as the American Academy of Family Physicians, the American College of Cardiology, the American College of Physicians, the American Pain Society, and the American Society of Anesthesiologists; health maintenance organizations such as the Harvard Community Health Plan; or consultative organizations such as the Rand Corporation have participated for years in the development of practice guidelines, treatment algorithms, and practice parameters. Newer initiatives are underway through the activities of the American Board of Medical Specialties, the American Medical Association, the Council of Medical Speciality Societies, among other academic and health services research entities.

For which clinical circumstances are guidelines warranted? This question has been approached by a variety of professional, third party, and regulatory groups. An aggregate overview table (Table 1) has been prepared by the Priority Setting Group, Council on Health Care Technology, of the IOM [13]. The primary and secondary criteria decided upon by the Priority Setting Group itself are also presented in Table 1. As an illustration of the results of topic selection, the first seven clinical practice guideline topics (of the 16 now under way) selected by the US Agency for Health Care Policy and Research (AHCPR) were:

- Visual impairment due to cataracts in the aging eye
- Diagnosis and treatment of benign prostatic hyperplasia
- Pain management
- Diagnosis and treatment of depressed outpatients in primary care settings
- Delivery of comprehensive care in sickle cell disease
- Prediction, prevention, and early treatment of pressure sores in adults
- Urinary incontinence in the adult

A guideline is successful if it improves practice; the guideline's educational content is only one part of this larger process [14]. Other parts include guideline dissemination and adoption of guideline recommendations into the realm of quality assurance and other review procedures. Concerning the guideline process itself, based upon IOM recommendations the AHCPR has set forth eight attributes of good guidelines [7]. These are:

- *Validity:* Practice guidelines are valid if, when followed, they lead to the health and cost outcomes projected for them, other things being equal. A prospective assessment of validity will consider the projected health outcomes and costs of alternative courses of action, the relationship between the evidence and recommendations, the substance and quality of the scientific and clinical evidence cited, and the means used to evaluate the evidence.
- *Reliability/Reproducibility:* Practice guidelines are reliable and reproducible

Table 1. (From [13])

Source	Criteria listed	Relation to Council on Health Care Technology criteria	
		Primary	Secondary
ACP	1. "Potential for significant health benefit" 2. "Potential for risk" 3. "Potential for wide application" 4. "Degree of interest to practitioners"	Individual patient outcome: explicit Patient population: explicit Cost: not included Variations: not included	Social/ethical: not included Medical knowledge: implied Policy impact: not included Assessment capacity: not included Feasibility: not included
AHA	1. "Importance to hospital management, especially their impact on costs" 2. "Perceived needs of hospitals"	Individual patient outcome: implied Patient population: implied Cost: explicit Variations: not included	Social/ethical: not included Medical knowledge: implied Policy impact: not included Assessment capacity: not included Feasibility: not included
AMA	1. "Potential impact on substantial patient population" 2. "Controversial within the medical community" 3. "Scientific data available to support evaluation"	Individual patient outcome: implied Patient population: explicit Cost: not included Variations: not included	Social/ethical: not included Medical knowledge: implied Policy impact: not included Assessment capacity: not included Feasibility: explit
BCBS	1. "Need to make financial coverage decisions"	Individual patient outcome: implied Patient population: implied Cost: implied Variations: implied	Social/ethical: not included Medical knowledge: not included Policy impact: explicit Assessment capacity: not included Feasibility: not included
IHPA	1. "Potential impact on patient outcome: safety and effectiveness" 2. "Prevalence of the condition" 3. "Variations in use" 4. "Existence of alternative technologies" 5. "Economic issues" 6. "Ethical and legal issues" 7. "Level of public/professional demand"	Individual patient outcome: explicit Patient population: explicit Cost: explicit Variations: explicit	Social/ethical: explicit Medical knowledge: implied Policy impact: implied Assessment capacity: not included Feasibility: not included

Table 1. (Part 2)

Source	Criteria listed	Relation to Council on Health Care Technology criteria	
		Primary	Secondary
IOM/ HCFA	1. "Burden of the illness" 2. "High prevalence of the illness in the Medicare population" 3. "High costs to the Medicare program" 4. "Substantial variation across geographic areas" 5. "High level of controversy regarding the alternative strategies for managing the condition" 6. "Availability of data to address the effectiveness questions"	Individual patient outcome: explicit Patient population: explicit Cost: explicit Variations: explicit	Social/ethical: not included Medical knowledge: implied Policy impact: implied Assessment capacity: not included Feasibility: explicit
NCHSR/ POARP	1. "Benefits and risks to the patient" 2. "Amount of unexplained variation in medical practice" 3. "Volumes of cases and treatments" 4. "Cost/charge per treatment" 5. "Sufficient data for analysis" 6. "Importance of the problem to the population"	Individual patient outcome: explicit Patient population explicit Cost: explicit Variations: explicit	Social/ethical: not included Medical knowledge: not included Policy impact: implied Assessment capacity: not included Feasibility: explicit
NIH/ OMAR	1. "Subject should have public health importance" 2. "Topic should affect a significant number of people" 3. "There should be a scientific controversy that would be clarified" 4. "Topic must have an adequately defined and available base of scientific information" 5. "The topic should be amenable to clarification on technical grounds" 6. "Health care cost impact" 7. "Preventive impact" 8. "Public interest" 9. "Timing of the conference should be such that it is likely to have a meaningful impact"	Individual patient outcome: implied Patient population: explicit Cost: explicit Variations: not included	Social/ethical: not included Medical knowledge: explicit Policy impact: explicit Assessment capacity: not included Feasibility: explicit

ACP, American College of Physicians; AHA, American Hospital Association; AMA, American Medical Association; BCBS, Blue Cross and Blue Shield; IHPA, Institute for Health Care Policy Analysis; Georgetown University; IOM/HCFA, Institute of Medicine Committee on Health Care Financing Administration; NCHSR/POARP, Patient Outcome Assessment Research Program (National Center for Health Services Research); NIH/OMAR, National Institutes of Health, Office of Medical Applications Research

1. if – given the same evidence and methods for guidelines development – another set of experts would produce essentially the same statements and
2. if – given the same circumstances – the guidelines are interpreted and applied consistently by practitioners or other appropriate parties.

A prospective assessment of reliability may consider the results of independent external reviews and pretests of the guidelines.

- *Clinical applicability:* Practice guidelines should be as inclusive of appropriately defined patient populations as scientific and clinical evidence and expert judgment permit, and they should explicitly state the populations to which statements apply.
- *Clinical flexibility:* Practice guidelines should identify the specifically known or generally expected exceptions to their recommendations.
- *Clarity:* Practice guidelines should use unambiguous language, define terms precisely, and use logical, easy-to-follow modes of presentation.
- *Multidisciplinary process:* Practice guidelines should be developed by a process that includes participation by representatives of key affected groups. Participation may include serving on panels that develop guidelines, providing evidence and viewpoints to the panels, and reviewing draft guidelines.
- *Scheduled review:* Practice guidelines should include statements about when they should be reviewed to determine whether revisions are warranted, given new clinical evidence or changing professional consensus.
- *Documentation:* The procedures followed in developing guidelines, the participants involved, the evidence used, the assumptions and the rationales accepted, and the analytic methods employed should be meticulously documented and described.

Cancer Pain Management Guidelines

Considering that the organized development of guidelines according to explicit and rigorous methods is a recent phenomenon, it is not surprising that clinically based groups have issued guidelines (not all of which are named such!) prepared according to different methods and issued to meet distinct needs of varied constituencies. If one excludes textbooks on cancer pain, or textbook chapters dealing with this topic, a sampling of the diverse collection of quasi-guidelines is presented in Table 2. In this broader context, the distinguishing features of the WHO publication for cancer pain relief are:

- Very broad targeting: worldwide, for different types of practitioners, both medical and nonmedical (e.g., nursing), in developed and undeveloped countries, and different types of settings (hospice, clinic, university hospital)

Table 2. A sample of existent guidelines on cancer pain management

Year	Reference	Title
1984	American Cancer Society [2]	The problem of nausea and vomiting in modern cancer chemotherapy
1986	World Health Organization [26]	Cancer pain relief
1986	American Cancer Society [3]	The treatment of pain in the patient with cancer
1986	Cleeland et al. [8]	A model for the treatment of cancer pain
1988	Australian National Health and Medical Research Council [25]	Management of severe pain
1989	American Pain Society [5]	Principles of analgesic use in the treatment of acute pain and chronic cancer pain. A concise guide to medical practice, 2nd edn.
1989	American Cancer Society [4]	Pain control in the patient with cancer
1990	Spross et al. [18]	Oncology Nursing Society position paper on cancer pain
1990	Wisconsin Cancer Pain Initiative [24]	Handbook of cancer pain management
1991	World Health Organization [27]	Cancer pain relief, 2nd edn.
1991	International Association of the Study of Pain, Task Force on Professional Education [11]	Core curriculum for professional education in pain
1991	Max et al. [15]	American Pain Society quality assurance standards for relief of acute pain and cancer pain

- Little explicit attention as to how the different roles of varied types of clinicians involved in multidisciplinary care can be best fitted together on a day-to-day level (e.g., social service or discharge planning in developed countries)
- No guidance as to how best to assure that this method for pain control is implemented within any particular socioeconomic framework (e.g., quality assurance or total quality management in developed countries); only general statements that may be correct but lack substance (e.g., "Governments should encourage health care workers to report to the appropriate authorities any instance in which oral opioids are not available for cancer patients who need them.")

- No information as to the precise relationship between the evidence cited and the construction of the recommendations: i.e., did the expert panel come to a consensus first, then cite references to support its view, or exhaustively review and synthesize the literature according to explicit search criteria, and on that basis form its recommendations?
- A deliberate and appropriate focus on a small number of standard oral medications, and away from invasive (e.g., neurosurgical) or technologically based approaches to pain relief (e.g., intraspinal catheters), even though economic progress in Europe and elsewhere (e.g., Asia) may foster the increased use of these modalities in selected cases.

Balanced against the above critique is the overwhelming strength of the document's simplicity of approach, emphasis upon therapeutic (oral or rectal) routes that are universally available, and its now documented success at relieving cancer-related pain in approximately 90% of patients treated according to its recommendations.

If one were to attempt to retain the successful aspects of the WHO document, yet address the points raised above, how might one best proceed in advancing the guideline process further? In the absence of any outcome-oriented studies that test the end result upon patient care and patient satisfaction of implementing one or another system of guideline development, and disseminating or otherwise propagating the resultant guideline products, these remarks must be heuristic and not based on specific data.

First, it is perhaps too general a target to aim for worldwide implementation of a treatment plan, given the vast differences in economic, social, and governmental conditions across the globe. Even regional geographic targets (e.g., Scandinavia, Western or Eastern Europe) may not share the same language or diagnostic classifications, or systems of medical practice and the associated organization, regulation and economics. Hence a large-scale guideline effort might best be subdivided into national efforts, and then common points merged in subsequent stages. Second, within a narrower geographical or social context, day-to-day and longer term treatment goals could be defined explicitly (e.g., reduction of pain intensity by a certain percentage, or worst pain intensity no higher than a certain limit). Such definition allows these performance standards to be fitted into institutional quality assurance and related review procedures, in order to sustain their effectiveness and consistency independent of the vagaries of individuals and their varying motivation levels. Third, assignment of individual or institutional responsibility for surveying and attaining explicit pain treatment outcomes must be a part of the guideline. Fourth, multiple peer reviewers and testing sites should be involved in the pre-release testing and validation of the guidelines, rather than leaving it to such interested individuals as come forth to perform validation studies in the post-release phase. Fifth, an a priori decision should be made concerning the specific literatures (languages, disciplines, study design etc.) to be examined for data relevant to the guideline, and clear procedures established for gathering and synthesizing such information in the guideline context. Lastly, careful country- and context-specific plans must be set in place for dissemination of guidelines through educational, medical review, and other channels, and these should be coupled with monitoring to assess the impact, if any, of guideline dissemination and implementation upon clinical practice.

The above thumbnail sketch of the content and context of the WHO guideline for cancer pain management is presented with the goal of evoking discussion to refine planning for and management of the continued evolution of this uniquely influential document. It may be that no additional clinical gains will accrue if the development process for this document becomes more formalized; nonetheless, it is difficult to see how formalization can be avoided if the patient outcomes implicit in this document are to become an integral and monitored part of clinical care, reimbursement, quality assurance, and institutional accreditation.

References

1. American Cancer Society (1992) Cancer facts and figures – 1992. American Cancer Society. Atlanta
2. American Cancer Society, Durant JR (1984) The problem of nausea and vomiting in modern cancer chemotherapy. American Cancer Society, New York (Professional education publication)
3. American Cancer Society, Foley KM (1986) The treatment of pain in the patient with cancer. American Cancer Society, New York (Professional education publication)
4. American Cancer Society, Hill CS, Portenoy RK (1989) Pain control in the patient with cancer. American Cancer Society, Atlanta (Professional education publication)
5. American Pain Society (1989) Principles of analgesic use in the treatment of acute pain and chronic cancer pain. A concise guide to medical practice, 2nd edn. American Pain Society, Skokie, IL
6. Bonica JJ (1984) Treatment of cancer pain: current status and future needs. Pain 2:196
7. Carr DB, Jacox A (1991) Pain management guidelines: a status report. ASA Newsletter (April) 55:12–16
8. Cleeland CS, Rotondi A, Brechner T, Levin A, MacDonald N, Portenoy R, Schutta H, McEniry (1986) A model for the treatment of cancer pain. J Pain Symptom Manage 1:209–215
9. Daut RL, Cleeland CS (1982) The prevalence and severity of pain in cancer. Cancer 50:1913–1918
10. Field MJ, Lohr KN (eds) (1990) Clinical practice guidelines. Directions for a new program. National Academy Press, Washington
11. Fields HL (ed) (1991) CORE curriculum for professional education in pain. International Association for the Study of Pain, Seattle
12. Grond S, Zech D, Schug SA, Lynch J, Lehmann KA (1991) Validation of World Health Organization guidelines for cancer pain relief during the last days and hours of life. J Pain Symptom Manage 6:411–422
13. Lara ME, Goodman C (eds) (1990) National priorities for the assessment of clinical conditions and medical technologies. Report of a pilot study. National Academy Press, Washington
14. Max MB (1990) Improving outcomes of analgesic treatments: is education enough? Ann Intern Med 113:885–889
15. Max MB, Donovan M, Portenoy RK, Cleeland CS, Ready LB, Carr DB, Edwards WT, Simmonds MA, Evans WO (1991) American Pain Society quality assurance

standards for relief of acute pain and cancer pain. In: Bond MR, Charlton JE, Woolf CJ (eds) Proceedings of the 6th world congress on pain. Elsevier, Amsterdam, pp 185–189
16. Schug SA, Zech D, Dörr U (1990) Cancer pain management according to WHO analgesic guidelines. J Pain Symptom Manage 5:27–32
17. Siraisi NG (1990) Medieval and early renaissance medicine. University of Chicago Press, Chicago
18. Spross JA, McGuire DB, Schmitt RM (1990) Oncology Nursing Society position paper on cancer pain. Oncol Nurs Forum 17:595–614, 751–760, 943–955
19. Swerdlow M (1989) The WHO concept of cancer pain relief. Schmerz Pain Douleur 10:130–133
20. Takeda F (1986) Results of field-testing in Japan of the WHO draft interim guidelines on relief of cancer pain. Pain Clin 1:83
21. Twycross RG, Fairfield S (1982) Pain in far-advanced cancer. Pain 14:303–310
22. Ventafridda V, Tamburini M, Caraceni A, DeConno F, Naldi F (1987) A validation study of the WHO method for cancer pain relief. Cancer 59:850–856
23. Walker VA, Hoskin PJ, Hanks GW, White ID (1988) Evaluation of WHO analgesic guidelines for cancer pain in a hospital-based palliative care unit. J Pain Symptom Manage 3:145
24. Weissman DE, Burchman SL, Dinndorf PA, Dahl JL (1990) Handbook of cancer pain management, 2nd edn. Wisconsin Cancer Pain Initiative
25. Working Party on Management of Severe Pain (1988) Management of severe pain. National Health and Medical Research Council, Australian Government Publishing Service, Canberra
26. World Health Organization (1986) Cancer pain relief. WHO, Geneva
27. World Health Organization (1991) Cancer pain relief, 2nd edn, Annex 1. World Health Organization, Geneva

Systemic Opiate Treatment

Uwe Dethlefsen

Pain is the most frequent reason for a patient to visit his physician. The patient's greatest fear when confronted with cancer is the accentuated potential for pain. Effective treatment of chronic pain has existed for years [5, 14] but, due to side effects and still existing myths, many physicians at times are unable to control a patient's pain effectively [7]. Pain is a major symptom in 70% of patients with far-advanced cancer, and it continues to be the case that the majority of patients do not receive satisfactory pain relief. Reasons for this include a lack of awareness that established methods already exist for managing cancer pain, and the failure to teach health care professionals systematically about pain management. We have to remember that every day more than 3.5 million people suffer from cancer pain, and only a few receive adequate treatment for it [4]. Therefore, we have repeatedly to call for these established therapeutic concepts to be put into practice in daily clinical routine, and not only reserved for a few pain clinics.

The WHO stepladder for cancer pain relief provides clear practical advice on the use of potent pain relief drugs and on the therapeutic strategies, rules and principles that need to be followed [15]. The key concept underlying the use of analgesics in cancer pain management is "by the clock and by the ladder." Thus, drugs should be given on a regular basis by the clock only. The next dose should be given before the effects of the previous one has fully worn off; in this way it is possible to relieve pain continously. Administration on demand should be avoided as this cannot relieve persistent pain and thus erase the patient's memory and fear of pain. The dose of an analgesic has to be individualized and should be titrated against the patient's pain. It should be increased gradually until the patient feels comfortable. If one drug is not effective enough, another, stronger one should be prescribed according to the WHO step plan.

The WHO step plan is a clinical approach to drug treatment of patients with chronic cancer-related pain:

1. Start with a non-narcotic analgesic every 4–6 h and remember that non-narcotic analgesics have a ceiling effect. For aspirin this is usually about 1300 mg/dose; increasing the dose beyond this amount will not increase the analgesic effect.

Table 1. Differences in the treatment of acute and chronic pain. (From [13])

	Acute pain: pain relief	Chronic pain: pain prevention
Rapid onset of effect	Important	Seldom required
Administration method	Parenteral	Oral
Sedation	Often desired	Mainly undesired
Dosage	Mostly standardized	Individualized
Administration routine	On demand	By the clock at fixed intervals
Adjuvants	Seldom required	Often required

2. If additional analgesia is required, a weak narcotic agonist such as dihydrocodeine is added. Dihydrocodeine, does not have a ceiling effect, but doses higher than 240 mg/day can be limited by side effects such as nausea and constipation.
3. If more analgesia is required, a stronger narcotic such as morphine has to be used.

It must always be remembered that the choice and the dose of analgesics is determined by the severity of pain, and that treatments of acute and chronic pain are substantially different (Table 1).

In principle, there are enough drugs for effective treatment of cancer pain according to the second step of the WHO plan. However, the widespread lack of knowledge about their indication and, especially, their pharmacologic and pharmacokinetic properties needs to be made good by proper repeated education. The half-life of most weak opioid analgesics requires short dosage intervals and they are not comfortable for the patients.

Dihydrocodeine has an established place in the treatment of moderate to severe pain in a variety of conditions ranging from post-operative pain to arthritis and even cancer. Its efficacy in comparison to other analgesic preparations is well established.

The short half-life of dihydrocodeine in the body, when given as a conventional release tablet, necessitates administration as often as every 4 h, causing problems like breakthrough pain, disturbances of sleep and the inconvenience of having to remember to take tablets every 4 h. The development of slow-release formulations of dihydrocodeine is one example of an effective use of pharmaceutical science to improve the utility of an established drug. The controlled-release formulation of dihydrocodeine was designed to avoid the adverse effect associated with high peak dihydrocodeine plasma levels and to reduce the frequency of administration.

The results of pharmacokinetic studies confirm the controlled-release characteristics of dihydrocodeine slow-release tablets and provide additional evidence that a twice-a-day preparation of dihydrocodeine has been developed which meets the requirements for successful by-the-clock treatment of chronic pain in cancer patients [3]. Pain treatment with dihydrocodeine slow-release tablets given every 12 h, permits uninterrupted sleep and freedom from pain throughout the day and night in patients with moderately severe cancer pain.

In three different clinical trials the efficacy and safety of long-term systemic treatment with one or two dihydrocodeine slow-release tablets containing 60 mg dihydrocodeine given 12-hourly were examined in more than 100 in- and outpatients suffering from moderately severe cancer pain [1, 6, 10]. In these clinical studies pain scores and sedation scores were assessed 2-hourly using visual analogue scales. In all centres the visual analogue scores showed a clinically and statistically significant reduction of pain without sedation during treatment. After 2 weeks most of the patients suffered from no or only minor pain and no discomfort. The Karnofsky Index as a measure of patient's performance improved during treatment, underlining the fact that pain relief enhances quality of life. These results clearly show how necessary it is that guidelines, like the WHO step plan, become more widely used.

When weak opioids like codeine and dihydrocodeine were given orally in the range of 30–120 mg/dose in combination with a non-opioid drug, preferably at 12-h dose intervals, the most common side effect during treatment was constipation, which was effectively treated by laxatives. During long-term treatment no signs of respiratory depression were seen, as pain is the physiological antagonist of the depressant effect of opioids. Other side effects were not a problem and no undexpected adverse reactions or physical dependence was reported. Cough suppression was a side effect of special benefit to the patients with bronchial carcinoma, since cough aggravates the intensity of pain. Comparing side effects with those of other centrally acting analgesics, dizziness and nausea occurred less often, which may be due to the slow-release mechanism of administration.

"As required" medication has no place in the treatment of persistent chronic pain, dihydrocodeine slow-release tablets given 12-hourly meet the requirements for a weak opioid analgesic in the second step of the WHO step plan, since these tablets can be given by the clock, each before the effect of the last has worn off and before the patient may think it necessary. Clinical experience and studies indicate that dihydrocodeine is a WHO second-step analgesic agent whose analgesic potency is higher than that of codeine and lower than that of morphine.

Extensive experience in effective pain control has shown that it is appropriate to use only one drug for each step of the analgesic ladder. If the drug of choice on either of the first two steps of the ladder is no longer effective, it is advisable to proceed up a step rather than try an alternative at the same level.

Therefore, should pain persist or increase, strong opioids like buprenorphine and morphine are to be given orally. These two drugs are virtually identical with regard to pain control and toxicity. One major difference is that buprenorphine has a ceiling effect, which is not know for morphine. Due to the pharmacological properties of buprenorphine, is has to be given

6- to 8-hourly. These time intervals are acceptable for the treatment of chronic cancer pain. Conventional morphine solutions have to be given 4-hourly and are in general not recommended for the treatment of chronic cancer pain. Generally speaking, morphine is the strong opioid of choice. Contrary to popular belief, most patients do not require large doses of morphine. According to clinical studies, 67% of patients need more than 30 mg, 91% need less than 100 mg and only 2% need more than 200 mg at 4-hourly intervals.

The pharmacokinetics of morphine have been widely misunderstood. Because of the first-pass metabolic process, only 30–40% of an orally administered dose actually enters the systemic circulation. The ratio of morphine required when given parenterally compared to orally is about 1:3 after repeated doses. The half-life of most third-step analgesic requires administration intervals which are insufficient for adequate treatment of chronic cancer pain. With modern galenical technology, morphine slow-release tablets have been developed to maintain plasma levels within a therapeutically effective range for 12 h. Twice-daily administration of morphine shows in steady state a peak-to-trough variation which reduces the possible side effects of high plasma levels and breakthrough of pain at low plasma levels [12].

It has to be borne in mind that morphine slow-release tablets cannot be used to treat acute pain or an acute exacerbation of chronic pain, because there is a delay of 2–4 h before peak plasma level concentrations are achieved. For this reason, it is always advisable to use aqueous morphine solutions when adjusting the dose to find the effective level for any individual patient. For the dosage interval of 12 h, three times the dose of the morphine solution has to be given as a morphine slow-release tablet. This regimen is suitable for patients on a stable dosage of morphine for whom a twice- or thrice-daily regimen would be preferable and may be substituted for aqueous morphine solutions in equivalent doses. Usually twice-daily administration is sufficient, although some patients need to take morphine slow-release tablets three times daily [e.g. 2, 8, 11, 16].

In clinical studies proof was obtained that the analgesic effect of morphine slow-release tablets given 12-hourly was equivalent to that of morphine solutions. From various clinical studies it can be concluded, when comparing pain scores during treatment with morphine slow-release tablets, that baseline scores for pain, anxiety, mood and sedation indicate that morphine slow-release tablets given 12-hourly are as effective as 4-hourly aqueous solutions. The individual twice-daily dose allows escape from the "vicious circle" of pain, anxiety, depression and insomnia.

The most troublesome side effects of opioids are drowsiness, constipation, nausea and vomiting. Drowsiness is usually only a problem at the start of treatment with morphine, and some explanation to the patients will help them to cope with it. Part of this drowsiness and sleepiness is due to the fact that the patient may be having a first good sleep after weeks or months of pain or pain-disturbed nights. We have to remember that no patient on long-term treatment with opioids would accept being painfree if this also means being sedated as well. If sedation is seen even after some days of treatment, this may be a sign that opioids are contraindicated.

Alertness is not depressed when morphine is given for opioid-sensitive cancer pain: indeed, the mental and physical performance of patients with pain increases when opioids are effective against their pain. Proof of this was given by testing reaction times of patients before and after instituting morphine therapy [9]. Most patients return to their former occupation when morphine therapy has freed them from pain.

At the beginning of treatment with morphine some patients may complain of nausea and vomiting, but this effect usually passes in a few days. Antiemetics should be used liberally if nausea and vomiting persist, but 30–50% of patients taking morphine never experience these side effects.

Fear of respiratory depression is usually one of the reasons for not giving opioids when they are properly indicated. Respiratory depression is not a problem in cancer patients receiving oral opioids. As long as the patient has pain the dose of the narcotic can safely be titrated against the pain until control is achieved.

Myths and fears of addiction associated with the therapeutic use of strong opioid analgesics have been a major impediment to the use of these drugs. It is encouraging to find that much has been done over the last 30 years to demonstrate that these fears are unfounded and irrelevant to the use of oral morphine in cancer pain. Several published studies demonstrate that long-term morphine treatment results in a slower rate of increasing the dose as well as a longer period without an increase at all. It is generally accepted that, when morphine is given within the context of comprehensive and continuing care, it can be used for long periods in cancer patients without concern about tolerance. It must be emphasized repeatedly that, in practice, the main reason for increasing the dose has not been tolerance but progression of the disease.

To summarize: analgesia should be kept simple and an adequate dose should be given at regular intervals so that the pain is suppressed and its memory eradicated, since for the cancer patient the pain is a constant reminder that the illness may be incurable. Successful treatment resulting in pain relief must include explanations and reassurance leading to understanding and hope which, too, have an important analgesic effect. The individual twice-daily dose of dihydrocodeine and morphine slow-release tablets allows an escape from the vicious circle of cancer pain; patients become more independant of their physicians and have the chance of reintegrating themselves in their family and their usual environment with a reasonable quality of life. This is the reason that modern galenical technology has given the opportunity for a renaissance of morphine and dihydrocodeine.

References

1. Ammon J, Andreopoulos D, Karstens JH (1989) Dihydrocodein-Retardtabletten (DHC) – Wirksamkeit bei Tumorpatienten. In: Dethlefsen U (ed) Chronischer Schmerz – Therapiekonzepte. Springer, Berlin Heidelberg New York, p 97
2. Bates TD, Kearney MK (1987) Longer-term control of pain in terminal cancer with MST continus tablets. In: Doyle D (ed) 1986 International symposium on pain control. Royal Society of Medicine Services, London, p 5
3. Dethlefsen U (1989) Chronischer Schmerz und Pharmakokinetik. In: Dethlefsen U (ed) Chronischer Schmerz – Therapiekonzepte. Springer, Berlin Heidelberg New York, p 76
4. Diekmann JM, Engber D, Wassem R (1989) Cancer pain control: one state's experience. Oncol Nurs Forum 16:219–223
5. Evans PJD (1983) Opiates in the management of chronic pain. Clin Anesthesiol 1:71–94
6. Gatzemeier U, Groth G, Munski T (1989) Verbesserung der Lebensqualität bei Patienten mit fortgeschrittenem Bronchialcarcinom durch optimierte Schmerztherapie mit Dihydrocodein-Retardtabletten (DHC). In: Dethlefsen U (ed) Chronischer Schmerz – Therapiekonzepte. Springer, Berlin Heidelberg New York, p 90
7. Hanks GW (1989) Oral morphine in cancer pain: fact and fiction. In: Twycross RG (ed) The Edinburgh symposium on pain control and medical education. Royal Society of Medicine Services, London, p 39
8. Hanks GW, Twycross RG, Bliss JM (1987) Controlled-release morphine tablets: a double-blind trial in patients with advanced cancer. Anaesthesia 42:840–844
9. Hartmann N, Zenz M (1986) Opiate und Fahrtüchtigkeit, In: Doenicke A (ed) Schmerz – Eine interdisziplinäre Herausforderung. Springer, Berlin Heidelberg New York, p 160
10. Hoffmann L, Sieker S, von Klinggräff G (1989) Dihydrocodein im Stufenplan der medikamentösen Schmerztherapie. In: Dethlefsen U (ed) Chronischer Schmerz – Therapiekonzepte. Springer, Berlin Heidelberg New York, p 83
11. Meed SD, Kleinman PM, Kantor TG, Blum RH, Savartese JJ (1987) Management of cancer pain with oral controlled-release morphine sulfate. J Clin Pharmacol 27:155–161
12. Sloan PA, Boos G, Thirlwell M, Maroun J, Besner JG, Mount B (1987) The steady-state pharmacokinetics of sustained-release morphine tablets (MST Continus) and oral morphine solution. In: Doyle D (ed) 1986 International symposium on pain control. Royal Society of Medicine Services, London, p 13
13. Twycross RG (1978) Relief of pain. In: Arnold E (ed) The management of terminal disease. Saunders, Philadelphia, p 65
14. Twycross RG, Zenz M (1983) Die Anwendung von oralem Morphin bei inkurablen Schmerzen. Anaesthesist 32:279–283
15. World Health Organisation (1986) Cancer pain relief. WHO, Geneva
16. Zenz M, Strumpf M, Tryba M, Röhrs E, Steffmann B (1989) Retardiertes Morphin zur Langzeittherapie schwerer Tumorschmerzen. Dtsch Med Wochenschr 114:43–47

Spinal Opioid Treatment for Chronic Pain: An Update

JOACHIM CHRUBASIK and SIGRUN CHRUBASIK

Spinal (epidural, intrathecal) administration of opioids is an alternative method for the management of intractable pain [19]. A nation-wide survey in Sweden reviewing 768 patients over 124 days suggests that the method has now been accepted as an outstanding method for treatment of certain chronic pain states, especially those due to malignancy [4]. Unfortunately, the quality of pain relief under the epidural or intrathecal opioid treatment was not recorded in these patients, except in those suffering from non-malignant pain. Only 7 out of 13 patients reported excellent or good pain relief with long-term epidural morphine, in a single case even up to 6 months [4].

A review of the literature confirms that spinal opioid administration does not always result in excellent pain relief. Although in the majority of patients at least some relief of pain was achieved, the quality of analgesia was poor in 363 out of 1201 patients under epidural morphine or buprenorphine (Table 1) and 103 out of 362 patients under intrathecal morphine (Table 2).

Table 1. Success rate of epidural opiate treatment

Number of patients CCP/CNMP (n)	Excellent or adequate pain relief (n)	Duration of treatment (days)[a]	Ref.
114/36	81	49 (7–397)	[8]
94/11	70	65 (7–283)	[22]
225/0	133	47 (7–420)	[25]
145/83	155	48 (7–443)	[29]
24/20	18/12	54/19 (6–129/3–47)	[42]
284/11	256/5	96/155 (1–1215)/?	[52]
154/0	108	? (21–501)	[58]

CCP, Chronic cancer pain; CNMP, chronic non-malignant pain.
[a] Mean (range).

In light of the short mean observation periods of about 3 months under epidural morphine and 6 months under intrathecal morphine, the failure rate of spinal opioid treatment due to technical problems and adverse effects may even be higher with longer treatment periods. However, the review of the literature indicated that the patients scheduled for spinal therapy were not always selected according to defined criteria. We assume, therefore, that proper selection of patients may increase the success rate of long-term spinal opioid treatment.

Criteria for Patient Selection

Chronic pain has multidimensional origins. The pain history with regard to nature, origin, and time pattern of the pain should, therefore, clearly indicate wheter the patient's pain may respond to spinal opioids [3]. Many so-called neuropathic as well as psychogenic types of pain are non-nociceptive

Table 2. Success rate of intrathecal opiate treatment for chronic malignant and non-malignant pain

Number of patients (n)	Quality of Analgesia Excellent (n)	Good (n)	Poor (n)	Duration of Treatment	Ref.
62		46	16	Initial test	[63]
23	19	2	2	4.5 months (12–1500 days)	[6]
27	5	18	4	(1–13 months)	[22]
40	27	9	4	7 months (2–24 months)	[30]
12		3	9	6 months (up to 2 years)	[35]
35	17	11	7	5 months	[49]
17	15		2	147 days (6–961 days)	[52]
14	7	4	3	3 months (1–23 months)	[55]
53		28	25	46 days (1–231 days)	[59]
23		12	11	8 weeks (1–26 weeks	[60]
43[a]	28		15	(Within 2 years)	[5]
5[a]			5[a]	12 weeks	[21]
8[a]	4	4		21 months	[49]

[a] Non-malignant pain (all other malignant)

and opioid-insensitive phenomena [4]. Best responses to spinal opioid treatment may be expected when the pain is continuous and originates from deep somatic structures. Co-existing continuous visceral pain or intermittent somatic pain originating from a pathological fracture, for example, are less opioid-responsive. Cutaneous pain from ulcers and fistulas and intermittent pain due to intestinal obstruction are only occasionally relieved by spinal opioids [3]. Pain characterization can, however, be difficult, since nerve involvement in radiating cancer pain can only be objectified by neuropathic lesions, which may, however, develop gradually [54]. Distinction between visceral pain and the activation of somatic nerves close to the diseased organ may also be difficult [54]. Where it is uncertain whether spinal opioids provide sufficient pain relief, spinal placebo administration may help to clarify the situation.

The main criteria for selecting the spinal mode of opioid administration [62] include opioid-sensitive pain that is not relieved by conventional treatments (e.g. surgery or oral medication) and opioid-sensitive pain of such magnitude that it totally dominates the patient's life. Spinal opioids are an alternative to sytematic opioids if an increasing opioid dose requirement is resulting in intolerable side effects. Spinal opioids are an alternative to rhizotomy, chordotomy, and cerebral and spinal stimulations and may be considered when pretreatments with these techniques have been unsuccessful. The patient must consent to the spinal procedure and know about potential adverse effects and complications. Furthermore, the patient's physical status must allow implantation of the proposed narcotic delivery system. Important factors are anxiety and depression, which often have to be treated by pharmacological and/or psychological means in addition to proceeding with spinal analgesia.

Spinal administration of opioids is contraindicated when the patients suffer from opioid-insensitive pain or refuse this mode of treatment. Patients suffering from generalized sepsis or any infection at the proposed dermal site of implantation, and patients receiving anticoagulant therapy should also be excluded [62].

Choice of the Drug Delivery System

Calculation of the costs of spinal opioid therapy in 63 patients suffering from intractable cancer pain clearly demonstrated that this mode of therapy, although expensive in long-term use (daily costs about US$ 30.00), is justified by the alleviation of pain it brings [45]. Patients remain in better mental and physical control and need less external help due to the reduced opioid dose requirement. A careful choice of the drug delivery system according to the patient's life expectancy is necessary to keep the costs of treatment within a reasonable range.

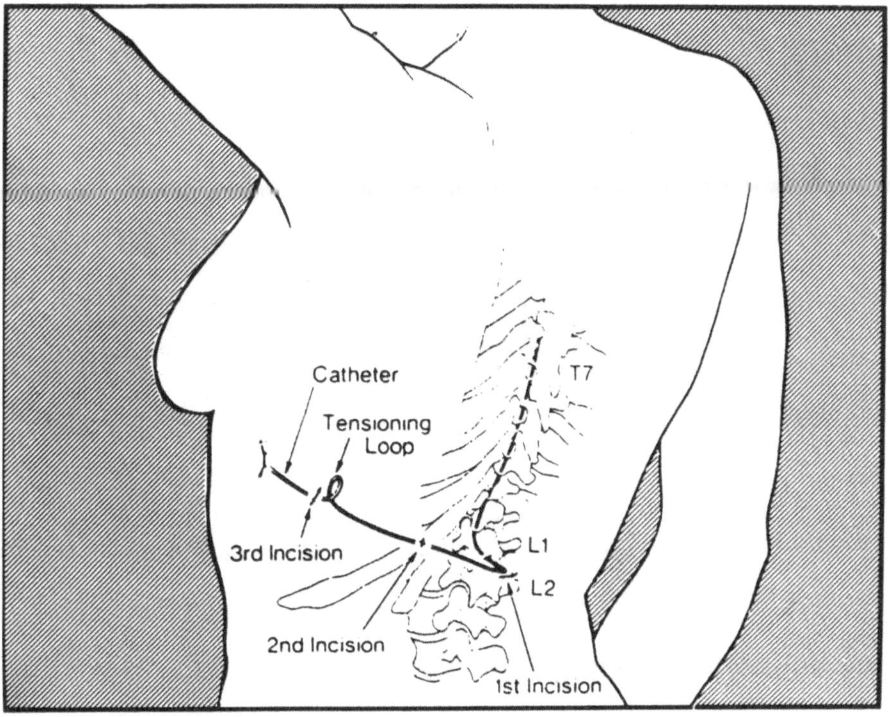

Fig. 1. A percutaneous catheter

Percutaneous Catheters

In short term care of intractable pain, percutaneous catheters (Fig. 1) offer the advantage of being inexpensive and simple to insert. However, the relatively high incidence of complications such as infection with long-term use, kinking, leakage, breakage, obstruction or displacement of the catheter limits their use for longer treatment periods. Bacterial filters connected to the epidural catheter help to prevent the introduction of infective organisms [9].

Subcutaneous Catheters

Subcutaneous tunnelling of the catheter laterally to the anterolateral chest wall or the iliac region helps to keep any local infection, which almost always ensues in this situation, sufficiently remote from the epidural space, and thus helps to prevent epidural sepsis [9]. Of 100 patients treated with subcutaneous catheters over an estimated mean period of 50 days, about 30% required more than one catheter [7]. Reasons for the change of extra-

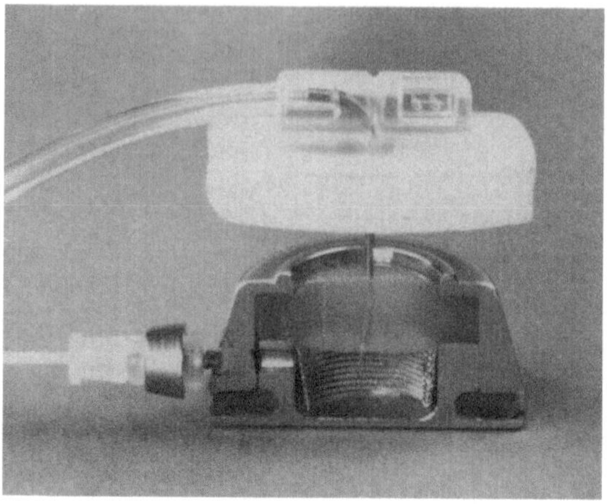

Fig. 2. An intrathecal catheter connected to a port system (cross sectional view). The opiate solution is injected by skin puncture into the port system, e.g. by means of a special needle (upper part of the figure).

dural catheters were leakage of LSF from the extradural space (7%), pain on injection (11%), functional disorders (5%) and infection in the tunnel (3%) [7].

Implantable Reservoirs

If patients have a life-expectancy of several months, the subcutaneous catheter should be connected to a subcutaneous injectable port system (Fig. 2). At present not only catheter technology but also that of portal systems need to be improved to reduce the incidence of complications. Basic requirements for implantable reservoirs are: to be easily palpable, easy to inject, relatively inexpensive and to survive at least 1000 injections via the skin [9]. In about 4% in one study, blockage of the portal system necessitated removal of the system [9].

Externally Portable Infusion Devices

An externally worn pump (Fig. 3) can be connected to the subcutaneous catheter or to the implanted reservoir by means of a special needle inserted through the skin [10]. This produces a largely closed circulation. The possibility of disconnecting the pump from the implanted reservoir grants the patients greater independence, for instance to shower, dress, etc.

There is a significant difference between the spinal infusion of opioids with constant flow rates and continuous, on-demand spinal opioid infusion. The latter offers the patient the possibilities of supplementary limited extra infusions on demand or of variation of the basal infusion rate according to the daily fluctuation in drug consumption or if tolerance develops [10]. Opioid consumption by continuous, on-demand epidural infusion is about

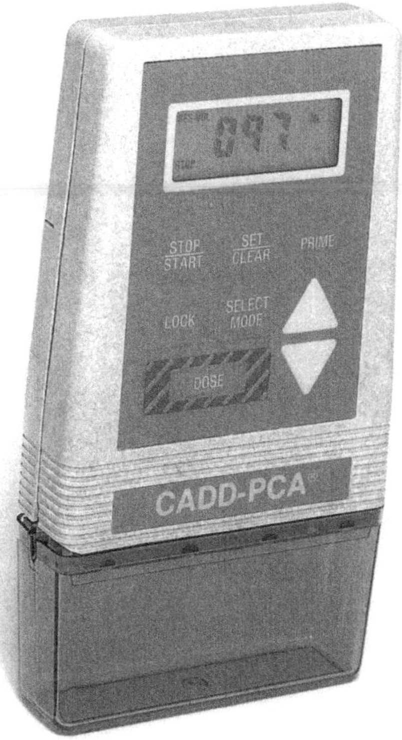

Fig. 3. An externally worn pump

30% lower than by infusion with constant basal rates [34]. Furthermore, a decrease in the drug demand can be recognized, and it is occasionally possible to return to oral medication [15].

Implantable Infusion Devices

The implantation of infusion devices (Fig. 4) is a considerable surgical procedure. However, implantable dosing devices, especially if they are programmable, are the most convenient in long-term treatment with spinal opioids. They offer a lower risk of complications than continuous opioid injection via the skin. Unfortunately, the high cost of the devices, which can only be employed once, limits the use of implantable dosing devices in patients with uncertain life expectancies. Technical development is required to facilitate refilling of these devices.

Description of the Implantation Technique

The placement of the spinal catheter may be carried out with the patient in the sitting, lateral or prone position. The position should be convenient for

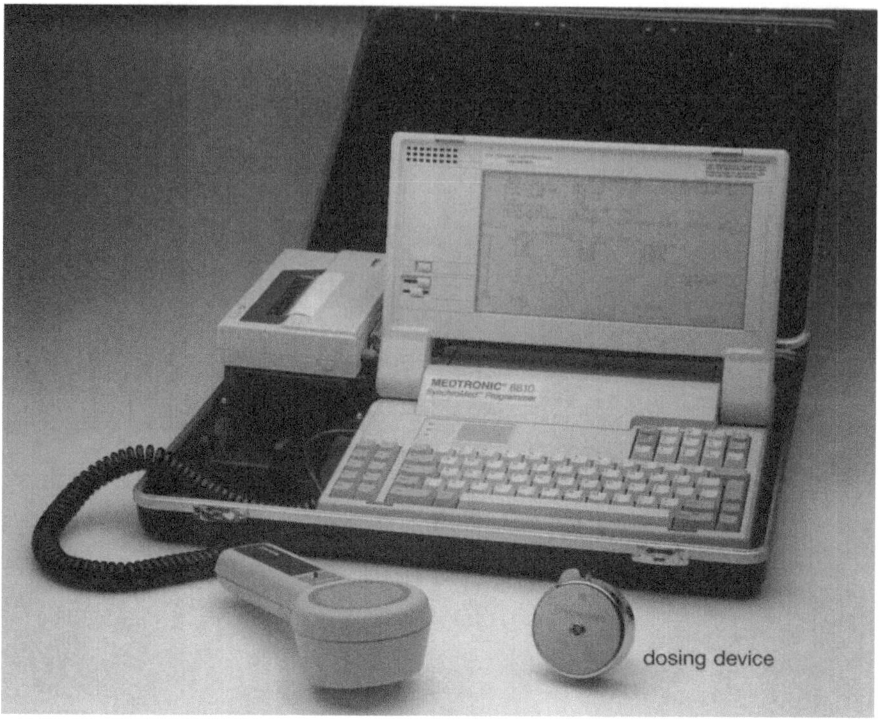

Fig. 4. An implantable dosing device with programmer

the patient for about 15–20 min when placing a subcutaneous catheter, for about 30 min more when a port system is implanted, and for at least about an hour for the implantation of an infusion device. If the staff are proficient in the method, the implantation time may even be shorter and require only minimal adjunctive narcotics or sedatives [61].

After aseptic preparation of the skin, including the tunnelling site and the catheter exit site, a Tuohy needle is placed, after infiltration with local anaesthetics and skin incision, into the spinal space at the desired lumbar or thoracic interspace. The catheter is then advanced through the Tuohy needle and placed several centimetres into the epidural or intrathecal space. Occcasionally it is easier to advance the catheter within the Tuohy needle after wetting both needle and catheter with saline [61]. After removal of the Tuohy needle, a tunnelling device of the desired lengths is advanced through the subcutaneous tissue from the desired catheter exit site incision to the incision site of the Tuohy needle after infiltration of the subcutaneous tissue with local anaesthetics. The tunnelling device is carefully withdrawn until the catheter tip is outside the skin. A subcutanous reservoir or an implantable infusion device may then be attached to the distal end of the catheter after making a small subcutanous pocket. The surgical procedure is completed in the usual way.

Considerations Prior to Implanting Any Drug Delivery System

Prior to implantation of a device for spinal opioid treatment, the following should be considered [62]:

1. The procedure, expected goals, and potential side-effects should be explained in detail to the patient and family.
2. The opioid and its dosage should be determined.
3. The daily epidural or intrathecal opioid consumption as well as subjective pain scores under the treatment, level of activity, amount of sleep, need for additional analgesics or centrally acting drugs (e.g. antidepressants), and the side effects under the treatment should be recorded.

Failure to clearly demonstrate efficacy of the spinal opioids during the preimplantation trial could result in the patients being subjected to implantation of a delivery system that fails to achieve pain relief [62]. There is evidence that concomitant spinal administration of local anaesthetics and opioids may be effective in the treatment of cancer pain refractory to spinal opioids alone [56].

Causes of Treatment Failure

Treatment may fail for several reasons [62]: spinal injection not made in the correct place; incorrect spinal opioid dosage or opioid-resistant pain; psychological reasons such as depression or use of pain as an attention-seeking device; advanced tolerance to opiates or physical dependence.

Choice of Opioid

Morphine

Hydrophilic morphine is characterized by a strong intrinsic analgesic activity. There are large discrepancies in the analgesia produced by a given morphine dose depending on how dose it is injected to the spinal cord. The epidural morphine dose requirement is about 10 times lower than the intravenous morphine dose requirement [18, 57], but exceeds the intrathecal morphine dose requirement by a factor of 10 [32]. Morphine is therefore an appropriate opioid for spinal treatment. The occurrence of respiratory depression due to morphine accumulation within the CSF is negligible [14] if morphine is continuously titrated into the epidural or intrathecal space [11].

Methadone

Although lipophilic methadone has a mμ opioid receptor affinity similar to morphine, its intrinsic analgesic activity is very weak. Relative to morphine, therefore, the closer methadone is placed to the spinal cord, the more methadone is required for analgesia: epidural methadone is only half as potent as epidural morphine [18, 24], while intrathecal methadone produced analgesia of inferior quality even at a dosage ten times higher than that of morphine [32, 33]. This and the fact that, due to its long terminal elimination time, no methadone is saved when changing from the intravenous [39] to the epidural route [24] of administration, make methadone inadvisable for intrathecal use.

Meperidine

Moderately lipophilic meperidine is characterized by a weak intrinsic analgesic activity. For epidural analgesia about 30 times more meperidine than morphine is required [12, 65]. Although its postoperative epidural dose requirement is not much lower than its intravenous dose requirement [57, 65], meperidine may be used as an alternative for morphine in spinal treatment.

Fentanyl

Due to the very high intrinisic analgesic activity of fentanyl, postoperatively a dosage 11 times lower than that of morphine suffices for analgesia at the epidural level [11]. Short-acting fentanyl may therefore be recommended for long-term spinal infusion treatment, although its intravenous-epidural dose discrepancy is far lower than that of morphine [18, 28].

Alfentanil

In contrast to fentanyl, alfentanil has a weak intrinsic analgesic activity. Although about four times more potent than morphine in postoperative intravenous treatment [2, 57], the two opioids are equipotent at the epidural level [18]. A comparison of the intrathecal dose requirements is not yet available. Short-acting alfentanil may be used as a substitute for fentanyl in spinal infusion treatment.

Buprenorphine

The partial opioid agonist buprenorphine is extremely lipophilic. A comparison of postoperative intravenous and epidural buprenorphine dose requirements indicated equal consumptions [16, 37]. This brings into question the epidural use of this opioid, which is about eight times more potent than morphine at the epidural level [11]. Although at present there are no data comparing intravenous and intrathecal buprenorphine dose requirements, it does not seem likely that buprenorphine is an appropriate opioid for intrathecal use.

Tramadol

Partial opioid agonist tramadol, a cyclohexane derivative, is not restricted by German law due to its very low drug abuse potential [53]. Its intrinsic analgesic potency [11] is very weak and results in high postoperative dose requirements. The fact that almost equal tramadol doses were required for postoperative intravenous [36, 38] and epidural pain treatment [17] argues against the spinal use of this opioid.

Side Effects and Complications

From the data in the literature (Tables 1 and 2) it is not possible to determine the number of patients suffering from side effects and complications under spinal opioid treatment. Probably all patients had some sort of side effects or complications during the brief mean period of 3 months (epidural) [22] and 6 months (intrathecal) [35].

Side effects that might occur under spinal opioid treatment are either dose-independent side effects or related to the opioid dose administered. Side effects that might occur irrespective of the opioid dose include urinary retention, pruritus, pain from bolus, transpiration, and, depending on lipophilicity, sedation [11]. Dose-dependent opioid side effects include the occurrence of nausea/emesis, dysphoria, euphoria, and central depression, e.g. major sedation, respiratory depression, hypotension, constipation, and tachyphylaxis.

Opioid-familiar patients show less respiratory depression and other side effects than opioid-naive patients [51]. Almost all patients need an increasing opioid dosage over time to control pain. A retrospective review of 163 patients by 19 physicians [64] revealed that patients suffering from pain of metastatic origin had a three-fold dosage over 3 months and a five-month increase over 6 months of intrathecal morphine treatment. Tolerance developed more quickly with bolus intrathecal injections than with continuous intrathecal infusions [55]. However, it may be difficult to distinguish tolerance from disease progression or the appearance or preeminence of a more morphine-resistent type of pain. Alternative spinal drugs may then be required to achieve sufficient pain relief.

Possible complications during spinal opioid therapy include mostly technical failures, such as mechanical device problems, leaking reservoir, catheter disconnection, dislocation, kinking, catheter, or port occlusion, infections (local infections or meningitis) or CSF leakage or persistent fistulas with spinal headache [8, 22, 29, 43].

Drug Alternatives for Spinal Pain Treatment

In cases of opioid tolerance, a variety of substances have been injected into the epidural or intrathecal space, e.g. D-ala-D-leu-enkephalin [20, 44], met-enkephalin [1], β-endorphin [46, 47], clonidine [20, 27], labetalol [40], lysin-acetylsalicylate [23, 48], calcitonin [15, 26] and somatostatin [13, 41] and its derivative octreotide [50]. Controlled studies must be undertaken to rule out neurotoxicity and to prove that spinal use of these substances as sole analgesics or in combination [31] may be of benefit to patients suffering from intractable pain.

Summary

More than 10 years have passed since spinal (epidural, intrathecal) opioid treatment was introduced for intractable cancer pain relief. A review of the literature reveals that the success rate of the method is far lower than previously believed, although in most of the patients at least some alleviation of pain is achieved. The success of spinal opioid treatment is dependent on careful patient selection. The pain must be opioid-sensitive and intractable. The patient's physical and mental status should be within the normal range. Spinal opioid treatment is only an alternative to other palliative treatments of pain that have a high incidence of side effects and complications. Selection of the administration device is dependent on the cost ratio in relation to the patient's life expectancy. The rank order of drug devices (less expensive to more expensive) is: percutaneous catheters, subcutaneous catheters, port systems, externally portable infusion devices and implantable infusion devices. Patient-controlled spinal analgesia with externally portable or implantable infusion devices offers independence for the patient and less work for doctors and nursing staff. The method is preferable to intermittant spinal opioid bolus injections or infusions with constant opioid infusion rates. Morphine has been shown to be the most appropriate opioid for patient-controlled spinal analgesia since its systemic/spinal dose discrepancy is far greater than that of other opioids. In case of opioid tolerance alternative drugs are available. However, controlled studies are required to rule out any neurotoxic effect of these agents and to prove their analgesic effectiveness.

References

1. Andersen HB, Jorgensen BC, Engquist A (1982) Epidural met-enkephalin (FK 33-824): a dose-effect study. Acta Anaesthesiol Scand 26:69–71
2. Andrews CJH, Robertson JA, Chapman JM (1985) Postoperative analgesia with intravenous infusion of alfentanil. Lancet 2:671
3. Arner S, Arner B (1985) Differential effects of epidural morphine in the treatment of cancer-related pain. Acta Anaesthesiol Scand 29:32–36
4. Arner S, Rawal N, Gustafsson LL (1988) Clinical experience of long-term treatment with epidural and intrathecal opioids – a nationwide survey. Acta Anaesthesiol Scand 32:253–259
5. Auld AW, Maki-Jokela A, Murdoch DM (1985) Intraspinal narcotic analgesia in the treatment of chronic pain. Spine 10:777–781
6. Brazenor GA (1987) Longterm intrathecal administration of morphine: a comparison of bolus injection via reservoir with continuous infusion by implanted pump. Neurosurgery 21:484–491

7. Carl P, Crawford ME, Ravlo O (1984) Fixation of extradural catheters by means of subcutaneous tissue tunnelling. Br J Anaesth 56:1369–1371
8. Carl P, Crawford ME, Ravlo O, Bach V (1986) Longterm treatment with epidural opiates. Anaesthesia 41:32–38
9. Cherry DA (1987) Drug delivery systems for epidural administration of opioids. Acta Anaesthesiol Scand 31 Suppl 85:54–59
10. Chrubasik J (1985) Zur spinalen Infusion von Opiaten und Somatostatin. Hygieneplan, Oberursel
11. Chrubasik J, Magora F (1990) Relative epidural analgesic potencies of opiates in treatment of postoperative pain. Anesth Analg 70 Suppl:S60
12. Chrubasik J, Wiemers K (1985) Continuous-plus-on-demand epidural infusion of morphine for postoperative pain relief by means of a small, externally worn infusion device. Anesthesiology 62:263–267
13. Chrubasik J, Meynadier J, Blond S, Scherpereel P, Ackerman E, Weinstock M, Bonath K, Cramer H, Wünsch E (1984) Somatostatin, a potent analgesic. Lancet 2:1208–1209
14. Chrubasik J, Scholler KL, Wiemers K, Weigel K, Friedrich G (1984) Low-dose infusion of morphine prevents respiratory depression. Lancet 1:793
15. Chrubasik J, Falke KF, Zindler M, Volk B, Blond S, Meynadier J (1986) Is calcitonin an analgesic agent? Pain 27:273–276
16. Chrubasik J, Vogel W, Trötschler, H, Farthmann EH (1987) Continuous-plus-on-demand epidural infusion of buprenorphine versus morphine in postoperative treatment of pain. Drug Res 37:361–363
17. Chrubasik J, Warth L, Wüst H, Bretschneider H, Schulte-Mönting J, Röher HD, Zindler M (1988) Wirksamkeit peridural applizierten Tramadols bei der Behandlung von Schmerzen nach abdominalchirurgischen Eingriffen. Schmerz Pain Douleur 9:12–18
18. Chrubasik J, Wüst H, Schulte-Mönting J, Thon K, Zindler M (1988) Relative analgesic potency of epidural fentanyl, alfentanil and morphine in treatment of postoperative pain. Anesthesiology 68:929–933
19. Coombs DW (1985) Continuous intraspinal morphine analgesia for relief on cancer pain, 1st edn. Shea, Cambridge, pp 1–29
20. Coombs DW, Saunders RL, Gaylor MS, Block AR, Colton T, Harbough R, Pageau MG, Mroz W (1983) Relief of continuous chronic pain by intraspinal narcotic infusion via an implanted reservoir. JAMA 250:2336–2339
21. Coombs DW, Saunders RL, Lachance D, Savage S, Ragnarsson TS, Jensen LE (1985) Intrathecal morphine tolerance: use of intrathecal clonidine, DADLE, and intraventricular morphine. Anesthesiology 62:358–363
22. Crawford ME, Andersen HB, Augustenborg G, Bay J, Beck O, Benveniste D, Larsen LB, Carl P, Djernes M, Eriksen J, Grell AM, Henriksen H, Johansen SH, Jorgensen HOK, Moller IW, Pedersen JEP, Ravlo O (1983) Pain treatment on outpatient basis utilizing extradural opiates. A Danish multicentre study comprising 105 patients. Pain 16:41–47
23. Devoghel JC (1983) Small intrathecal dose of lysin-acetylsalicylate relieves intractable pain in man. J Int Med Res 11:90–91
24. Eimerl D, Magora F, Shir Y, Chrubasik J (1986) Patient-controlled analgesia with epidural methadone by means of an external infusion pump. Schmerz Pain Douleur 7:156–160
25. Erdine S, Aldemir T (1991) Long-term results of peridural morphine in 225 patients. Pain 45:155–159
26. Fraioli F, Fabbri A, Gnessi L, Moretti C, Santoro C, Felici M (1982) Subarachnoid calcitonin for intolerable pain. Lancet 2:831
27. Glynn C, Dawson D, Sanders R (1988) A double-blind comparison between epidural morphine and epidural clonidine in patients with chronic non-cancer pain. Pain 34:123–128

28. Gourlay GK, Kowalski SR, Plummer JL, Cousins MJ, Armstrong PJ (1988) Fentanyl blood concentration – analgesic response relationship in the treatment of postoperative pain. Anesth Analg 67:329–337
29. Hegelund K, Nielsen FM (1983) Pain treatment of long term basis, with extradural opiates. Acta Anaesthesiol Scand 27 Suppl 78 (69)
30. Hernandez JLR, Padron FR, de VeraReyes JA (1986) Administration intratecallumbar de morfine en el tratamiento del dolor del cancer avanzado. Rev Esp Anaestesiol Reanim 33:253–256
31. Heyman JS, Vaught JL, Mosberg HL, Haaseth RC, Porreca F (1989) Modulation of mu-mediated antinociception by delta agonists in the mouse: selective potentiation of morphine and normorphine by (D-Pen-2,D-Pen-5)enkephalin. Eur J Pharmacol 165:1–10
32. Jacobson L, Chabal C, Brody MC, Ward RJ, Ireton RC (1989) Intrathecal methadone and morphine for postoperative analgesia:a comparison of the efficacy, duration, and side-effects. Anesthesiology 70:742–746
33. Jacobson L, Chabal C, Brody MC, Ward RJ (1989) Intrathecal methadone 5 mg and morphine 0.5 mg for postoperative analgesia: a comparison of the efficacy, duration and side-effects. Anesth Analg 68:S132
34. Jansen EC (1983) Morphine pumps in the epidural treatment of pain. Acta Anaesthesiol Scand Suppl 26 (68)
35. Krames ES, Gershow J, Glassberg A, Kenefick T, Lyons A, Taylor P, Wilkie D (1985) Continuous infusion of spinally administered narcotics for the relief of pain due to malignant disorders. Cancer 56:696–702
36. Lehmann KA, Jung C, Hoeckle W (1985) Tramadol und Pethidin zur postoperativen Schmerztherapie: Eine randomisierte Doppelblinduntersuchung unter den Bedingungen der intravenösen On-Demand-Analgesie. Schmerz Pain Douleur 6:88–100
37. Lehmann KA, Gördes B (1988) Postoperative On-demand Analgesie mit Buprenorphin. Anaesthesist 37:65–70
38. Lehmann KA, Brand-Stavroulaki, Dworzak H (1986) The influence of demand- and loading dose on the efficacy of postoperative patient-controlled analgesia with tramadol. Schmerz Pain Douleur 4:146–152
39. Lehmann KA, Abu-Shibika M, Horrichs-Haermeyer G (1990) Postoperative Schmerztherapie mit l-Methadon und Metamizol. Anasth Intensivther Notfallmed 25:152–159
40. Margaria E, Gagliardi M, Palieri L, Treves S, Fanzago E (1983) Analgesic effect of peridural labetalol in the treatment of cancer pain. Int J Clin Pharmacol Ther Toxicol 21:47–50
41. Meynadiere J, Chrubasik J, Dubar M, Wünsch E (1985) Intrathecal somatostin in two terminally ill patients. Pain 23:9–12
42. Michon F, Des Mesnards VG, Girard M, Fischler M, Vourc'h G (1985) Analgésie peridurale morphinique de longue duré en pathologie néoplasique et vasculaire. Cah Anesthesiol 33:39–42
43. Motsch J, Bleser W, Ismaily AJ, Distler L (1988) Kontinuierliche intrathekale Opiattherapie mit tragbaren Medikamentenpumpen bei Karzinomschmerzen. Anasth Intensivmed Notfallmed 23:271–275
44. Moulin DE, Inturrisi CE, Foley KM (1986) Cerebrospinal fluid pharmacokinetics of intrathecal morphine sulfate and D-Ala-D-Leu-Enkephalin. Ann Neurol 20:218–222
45. Mueller H, Lüben V, Zierski J, Hempelmann G (1988) Long term spinal opiate treatment. Acta Anesthesiol Belg 39 Suppl 2:83–86
46. Oyama T, Jin T, Yamaya R (1980) Profound analgesic effects of β-endorphin in man. Lancet 1:122–125
47. Oyama T, Fukushi S, Jin T (1982) Epidural β-endorphin in treatment of pain. Can Anaesth Soc J 29:24–26
48. Pellerin M, Hardy F, Abergel A, Boule D, Palacci JH, Babinet P, Wingtin NG, Glowinski J, Amiot JF, Mechali D, Colbert N, Starkman M (1987) Douleur chronique rebelle des cancereux. Presse Med 16:1465–1468

49. Penn RD, Paice JA (1987) Chronic intrathecal morphine for intractable pain. J Neurosurg 67:182–186
50. Penn RD, Paice JA, Kroin JS (1990) Intrathecal octreotide for cancer pain. Lancet 1:738
51. Pfeifer BL, Sernaker HL, Ter Horst UM (1988) Pain scores and ventilatory and circulatory sequelae of epidural morphine in cancer patients with and without prior narcotic therapy. Anesth Analg 67:838–842
52. Plummer JL, Cherry DA, Cousins MJ, Gourlay GK, Onley MM, Evans KHA (1991) Long-term spinal administration of morphine in cancer and non-cancer pain: a retrospective study. Pain 44:215–220
53. Richter W, Barth H, Flohe L, Giertz H (1985) Klinische Untersuchung zur Abhängigkeitsentwicklung bei oraler Therapie mit Tramadol. Drug Res 35:1742–1744
54. Samuelsson H, Hedner T (1991) Pain characterization in cancer patients and the analgesic response to epidural morphine. Pain 46:3–8
55. Shetter AG, Hadley MN, Wilkinson E (1986) Administration of intraspinal morphine sulfate for the treatment of intractable cancer pain. Neurosurgery 18:740–747
56. Sjöberg M, Appelgren L, Einsarsson S, Hultman E, Linder LE, Nitescu P, Curelaru I (1991) Long-term intrathecal morphine and bupivacaine in "refractory" cancer pain. I. Results from the first series of 52 patients. Acta Anaesthesiol Scand 35:30–43
57. Tamsen A, Hartvig P, Fagerlund C, Dahlström B, Bondesson U (1982) Patient-controlled analgesic therapy: clinical experience. Acta Anaesthesiol Scand Suppl 74:157–160
58. Tryba M, Zenz M, Strumpf M (1990) Long term epidural catheters in terminally ill patients – a prospective study of complications in 129 patients. Anesthesiology 73:A784
59. Ventafridda V, Spoldi E, Caraceni A, de Conno F (1987) Intraspinal morphine for cancer pain. Acta Anaesthesiol 31 Suppl 85:47–53
60. Verdenne JB, Esteve M, Guillaume A (1986) Injection de morphine intrathécale dans le traitement ambulatoire de la douleur néoplastique. J Chir (Paris) 123:330–332
61. Waldman SD (1987) A simplified approach to the subcutaneous placement of epidural catheters for long-term administration of morphine. J Pain Symptom Manage 2:163–166
62. Waldman SD, Feldstein GS, Allen ML, Turnage G (1986) Selection of patients for implantable intraspinal narcotic delivery systems. Anesth Analg 65:883–885
63. Wang JK (1985) Intrathecal morphine for intractable pain secondary to cancer of pelvic organs. Pain 21:99–102
64. Yaksh TL, Onofrio BM (1987) Retrospective consideration of the doses of morphine given intrathecally by chronic infusion in 163 patients by 10 physicians. Pain 31:211–223
65. Zaren B, Hartvig P, Tamsen A (1984) Patient-controlled analgesic therapy with epidural pethidine for postoperative pain relief. In: Wüst JH, Stanton-Hicks M, Zindler M (eds) Neue Aspekte in der Regionalanästhesie, Springer, Berlin Heidelberg New York, pp 173–176

Surgical Techniques in the Treatment of Pain

Y. LAZORTHES

Where medical therapy fails to ameliorate chronic irreductible pain, surgical intervention must be considered. One should not attempt to define a universal strategy, there being multiple forms of pain and just as many techniques. However, specialists agree that, although there is no one panacea, recipe or miracle cure, the approach should be selective and specifically adapted to the type of pain. Consequently, a choice of techniques is required. Using this approach, attitudes are modulated by personal experience and also by the availability of specialised techniques, e.g. microsurgery, stereotaxy and analgesic implants.

The idea of surgical intervention in pain therapy is not a new one. In the 16th century, Ambroise Paré transected sections of the superficial artery for the relief of migraine pain. In the 17th century the king's surgeon, Maréchal, performed trigeminal neurotomies for facial neuralgia. However, excepting these isolated attempts, the concept of surgical therapy in pain was born at the end of the 19th century with the publication of works by Horsley on the surgery of the trigeminal ganglion and by Abbé on posterior radicotomy.

So, can we speak today of pain surgery as defined by René Leriche [11] in 1940, now that needle, catheter and electrode have often replaced the scalpel in the operating theater? Neurosurgery is not the only possible mode of application of these techniques. The concept of surgery for pain has greatly evolved in recent years due to increasing knowledge of neurophysiological control mechanisms. This has quickly resulted in the development of new techniques in enhancing these intrinsic control mechanisms. Initially, based only on anatomical knowledge [4, 11, 20], cerebrospinal surgery only caused injury. Following recent developments in neurosurgery, interruptive surgery has been largely superseded by totally conservative methods such as neurostimulation, introduced in 1966 [5, 13, 14, 16, 17], and spinal opioids, first-used in 1977 [1, 2, 9, 21].

Surgical Techniques

There is currently a large repertory of analgesic surgical techniques. These can be roughly divided into two groups:

- Disruptive techniques, whereby the pain pathway is selectively sectioned
- Conservative techniques, whereby neurophysiological pain control mechanisms are reinforced

Neuroanatomical Methods

Techniques of Ascendent Pathway Interruption (Fig. 1)

Interruptions of the ascendent pathway are realised at peripheral or medullary sites because, at this level, the topography of the nociceptive pathways is well known and the nerve fibres or spinal pathways are well systematised, compact and relatively easy to access. Originally these were performed by direct surgical intervention with the naked eye under general anaesthesia. Since then, the use of microsurgical instruments, thermocoagulation and surgical CO_2 lasers has allowed for more precise intervention. The techniques of percutaneous neurolysis have developed to the point where it is done under stereotactic control under local anaesthetic. As the patient is conscious, precise neurophysiological determination of the target is possible. Based on a better understanding of the central nervous system (CNS), this is accomplished by sensitive neurostimulation coupled with motor stimulation, thereby decreasing the risk of injury to the adjacent motor pathways. Selective percutaneous thermocoagulation of the trigeminal ganglion, percutaneous cervical cordotomy and percutaneous posterior radicotomy are examples illustrating this method.

The neurolytic agents used are rarely chemical (pure alcohol, phenol, glycerol), as the extent of diffusion of chemical agents cannot be controlled. Normally, the neurolytic agent is thermal, generated at radiofrequency and connected to an active electrode which has a thermistor allowing precise temperature control and exactly delimited injury. Nociceptive fibres, being less protected, are more sensitive to coagulation and therefore, by progressive coagulation, it is possible to leave the large myelinated nerves undisturbed. Regardless of the technique or agent used, the interruption sites are chosen with regard to clinical type and area of pain. One must distinguish between peripheral and central techniques.

Figure 1 shows the available techniques from the periphery to the centre.

Peripheral Neurotomies

Peripheral neurotomy consists of interrupting the conduction of the nerve impulse between site of injury and entry into the CNS. While promising in theory, this technique has a very limited practical application because (a) the painful territory is rarely limited to the distribution of a single peripheral nerve, requiring multiple neurotomies with limited efficacy; (b) peripheral nerves are generally mixed and neurotomy can therefore lead to motor damage; and (c) section before the first spinal ganglion is generally followed

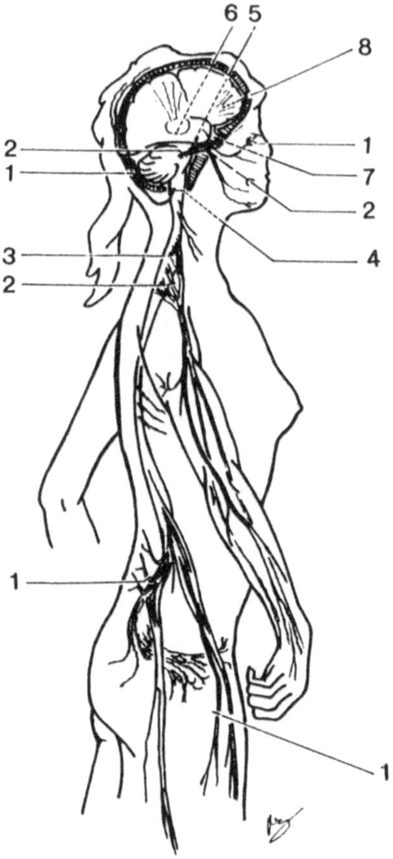

Fig. 1. Techniques of interruptions of the nociceptive pathways: *1* peripheral neurotomy; *2* posterior radicotomy; *3* lesion of the radiculomedullary junction; *4* upper cervical cordotomy; *5* mesencephalic tractotomy; *6* thalamotomy; *7* hypophysectomy; *8* frontal lobotomy

by nerve regeneration with consequent reemergence of pain. For these reasons, neurotomy or peripheral block has a very limited place in analgesic surgery. Percutaneous neurolysis is usually performed on:

1. The peripheral distribution of the trigeminal nerve in facial neuralgia
2. The posterior branch of C_2 in Arnold's neuralgia
3. The intercostal nerves (single or multiple) in intercostal neuralgia
4. The posterior branches of the lumbar spinal nerves by percutaneous thermocoagulation at the articular facets in chronic lumbar pain ("posterior branch syndrome")
5. The femoral cutaneous nerve at the level of the iliac spine in the corresponding neuralgia.

There are similarities between peripheral neurolysis and sympathectomies involving visceral sympathetic ganglia. Percutaneous or surgical sympathectomies, especially of the stellate ganglia in upper limb pain, coeliac ganglia in abdominal pain and splanchnic or lumbar ganglia in lower limb pain, were described by René Leriche, the pioneer of neurosurgery for pain. The actual indications for these sympathectomies are limited for the same reasons as in peripheral neurolysis.

Posterior Radicotomy (Fig. 2)

Posterior radicotomy consists of cutting the first sensory neuron on entry into the spinal ganglion prior to penetration into the spinal cord or the brainstem. Considered for a long time to be the simplest surgical intervention [4, 20], it is also the oldest. Proposed in 1889, its popularity increased greatly after World War II. It is based essentially on the fact that at the level of the posterior root all fibres are sensory and injury to them will be definitive. It does not expose one to motor disturbance. However, due to overlapping of dermatomes it must be extended to above and below the actual pain area. Therefore, in order to avoid extensive surgery, the indication is limited to cases of unilateral, clearly defined, delimited pain territories involving one nerve or maximally two adjacent nerves.

The posterior radicotomy of spinal nerves is commonly performed by open surgery, a small aperture being made in the spinal canal (laminectomy)

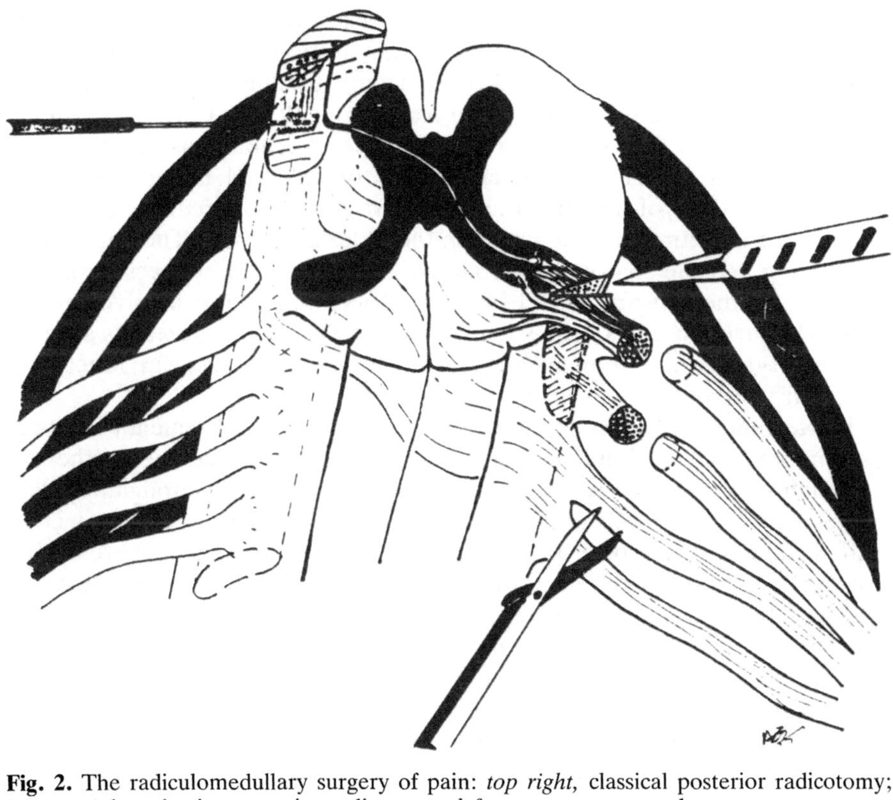

Fig. 2. The radiculomedullary surgery of pain: *top right,* classical posterior radicotomy; *bottom right,* selective posterior radicotomy; *left,* percutaneous cordotomy

using neurosurgical techniques. It can also be performed by percutaneous thermocoagulation.

Concerning cephalic pain, the most common indication is refractory trigeminal neuralgia. Neurotomy consists of cutting the ramus of the trigeminal nerve between the trigeminal ganglion and its penetration into the brainstem. Originally performed by Walter Dandy using open surgery, the technique has developed due to a better understanding of the sensory pathways and use of microsurgical techniques. However, the existence of dissociation of nerve fibres at the level of brainstem penetration means that selective neurotomy is permitted only where the painful territory is clearly defined and excludes risk to corneal sensibility and masticatory motor functions. Opinion swung in favour of pathophysiological hypotheses with regard to the triggering of such neuralgias. It is known that essential trigeminal neuralgia is due to abnormal contact of the nerve with the adjacent vascular supply, and lasting analgesia results only from obliteration of this supply. Other neurovascular pathologies, such as facial hemispasm, have led to the development of conservative microsurgical vascular decompression. Open surgical techniques are specialised interventions carrying the risk of damage to the cerebellopontine angle. Consequently, the percutaneous methods have a leading position, especially percutaneous thermocoagulation of the trigeminal ganglion (Fig. 3). First described by Sweet and Wepsic [18] in 1965, the technique consists of selective neurosection using controlled radiofrequency thermocoagulation following cutaneous puncture, advancing towards the trigeminal ganglion via the foramen ovale [6]. Carried out under brief general anaesthesia and rapidly reversible, percutaneous thermocoagulation is mildly invasive, relatively devoid of risk and is suitable for all patients regardless of health status. This last point is particularly important as this type of neuralgia is common in the older age group. The analgesia is longlasting and the sensory disturbances, such as tactile hypoaesthesia, are localised to the sensory branches of the trigeminal nerve involved in the pain. The procedure has been widely used and the long-term results are very satisfactory; there is a recurrence rate of 15% but one can repeat the procedure without increasing risk.

The technique of selective thermocoagulation by radiofrequency has been used in other cervical/cephalic neuralgias, notably the percutaneous thermocoagulation of the petrosal ganglion in glossopharyngeal neuralgia [7]. Posterior radicotomes, while only involving sensory pathways, are not selective, and section destroys both tactile sensory and thermosensory fibres. Neuroanatomical studies of the posterior fibres in the medulla oblongata, as reported by Sindou [15] have rendered it possible to differentiate between amyelinated (C) fibres and myelinated (A) fibres conducting tactile sensation. It is therefore possible, using a microsurgical technique, to selectively section at the anterior junction thereby making a selective radiculotomy.

This method is particulary important in upper limb neuralgias, where it is important for functional hand movement to preserve full sensory perception. It is also advocated in chronic pain due to sensory disafferentiation,

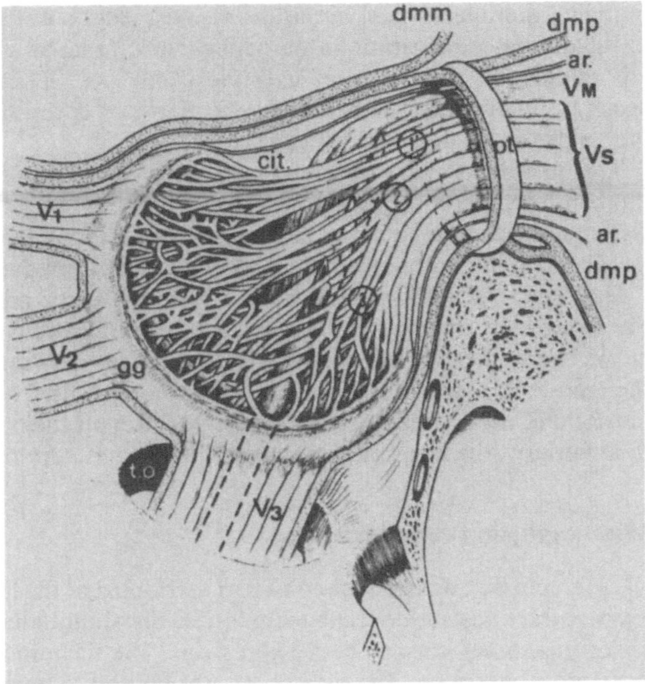

Fig. 3. Percutaneous thermocoagulation of the trigeminal ganglion: diagram showing the gangliocisternal complex and the penetration of the coagulation electrode. *dmm,* Dura mater of middle cerebral fossa; *dmp,* dura mater of posterior cerebral fossa; *ar.*, arachnoid; *VM,* motor trigeminal bundle; *VS,* sensory bundle; *cit.,* trigeminal cistern; *f.o.,* foramen ovale

where it is important to establish a balance between sensory "excitation" and medullary inhibition proximal to the level of the nerve lesion. This is the case in pain secondary to limb amputation and to shearing brachial plexus injury.

Anterolateral Cordotomy

Anterolateral cordotomy consists of section at the level of the spinal cord of the spinothalamic tract carrying the thermosensory fibres. Proposed in 1912 by Spiller and Martin [16], the technique lacked precision, having to be performed with the naked eye using open surgery [4, 20]. It was not until 1965 that it was further developed, when Rosomoff [12] reported the possibility of making a section at the cervical level with the accuracy of thermocoagulation (Fig. 3). Then, under local anaesthetic, with percutaneous puncture at the level of C1–2 and under radiological control, the target is identified by neurostimulation. This procedure makes it possible to accurately identify the nerves involving the pain territory. However, the mobility and anatomical variations of the medulla oblongata at the cervical level and the cooperation of the patient, who remains conscious throughout, all render this intervention extremely delicate. The target having been accurately detected, the ability of the operator determines the limitation of the analgesia to the pain-affected area.

The technique met with great success up to 1975, preceding the arrival of the conservative neurophysiological techniques. Until then, it was the most widely used technique and one can estimate the number of cases at approximately 2000 annually in the United States and Canada.

However, the indications were limited to unilateral pain distribution due to the major risk of respiratory and sphincter complications arising from bilateral nerve injury. On the other hand, as for classic open surgical cordotomies,in the long-term the pain had a tendency to reoccur after 1–2 years. Overall, the indications are limited to refractory pain of neoplastic origin and to unilateral distribution, which for all intents and purposes is very rare [6].

Mesencephalic Tractotomies

Mesencephalic tractotomies consist of sectioning at the level of the brainstem, by percutaneous stereotactic techniques, the spinothalamic bundle in which facial trigeminal sensory nerve fibres run. The technique is very precise and presents major risks. The indications are limited to pain of cancerous origin. The technique has been largely discontinued due to the development of local morphine therapy and is confined to very specialised centres.

Sensory Thalamotomy

It is at the level of the thalamus, the primordial sensory relay station, that neurosurgeons have long sought effective targets in the treatment of chronic pain, particularly since the introduction of stereotactic techniques. Areas of the thalamus can be selectively destroyed, provoking a corresponding contralateral anaesthesia. However, a major risk is that of accompanying "painful anaesthesia". These targets have been abandoned from the surgical point of view, but remain of interest in electrical neurostimulation analgesia.

Analgesic Hypophysectomy

Analgesic hypophysectomy consists of hypophyseal lysis using stereotactically controlled transnasal neurolytic agents (pure alcohol or thermocoagulation) [6]. The principle lies in the fact that refractory pain resulting from disseminated metastases of hormone-dependent cancers (prostate and breast) are ameliorated by the destruction of the hypophysis. Despite the fact that the technique is simple, due to the use of specific stereotactic measures developed by Talairach [19], it is very rarely indicated and has been superseded by local morphine therapy.

Methods of Activating Intrinsic Pain Control Mechanisms or Neurophysiological Control

These techniques are based on recent discoveries involving neuroelectrical and neurophysiological pain control mechanisms. They are divided into two groups; electrical neurostimulation and local, spinal or intraventricular morphine therapy.

Electrical Neurostimulation

Neurophysiological Basis and Principles [5, 6, 13, 14, 17]

The idea of using neuroelectrical stimulation is very old. As early as 46 B.C. Scriborius Largus used the electrical discharges of the light fish (40 V/100 Hz) to reduce the refractory pain associated with headache and gout. At the beginning of the 20th century the medical electrical therapy developed with the use of electrical currents of varying strengths with the aid of generators and various cutaneous electrodes. About 1950, scepticism and criticism ensured these methods were temporarily abandoned. It took the more recent work on neurophysiology and neurobiology coupled with the development of cardiac stimulators to bring about a renaissance in neurostimulation.

In 1959, Noordenbos, with his theory of a multisynaptic afferent system, showed the inhibitory affect of myelinated A fibres (tactile sense) on the amyelinated C fibres (temperature and pain sensitivity) at every synapse in the spinothalamic tract.

In 1965, Wall and Melzak proposed their gate control theory, based on the dual mechanism of metameric and central pain modulation. In this theory, pain sensation is conducted slowly by the small amyelinated C fibres, modulated in the gelatinous substance at the level of the posterior horns of the spinal cord by the long afferents from rapidly conducting myelinated A fibres. Therefore, stimulating these fibres enhances the inhibitory potential of the interneurons of the gelatinous substance and by so doing "closes the gate" on the pain impulse at the metameric level of entry as well as at all levels above. When the protective barrier is overridden by nociceptive stimuli, the "gate opens" and the perception of pain reoccurs. This theory, while fundamentally flawed, was valuable in renewing interest in analgesic electrical neurostimulation based on neurophysiological principles.

In 1966, Shealy and Mortimer, at the Harvey Cushing Society Congress, proposed that one could selectively stimulate the large-diameter myelinated afferent fibres and the first medullary synapse in chronic intractable pain.

In 1973, work by Liebeskind and de Besson confirmed the "morphine-like" action of the stimulation of periventricular and periaquaductal grey matter in the brainstem. The same inhibitory action on pain was demonstrated at the level of the third ventricle. The mechanism acts by reinforcing the central inhibitory affect by release of neurotransmitters involving the descending inhibitory system, which blocks nociceptive transmission distally.

Subsequently, numerous neurosurgeons reported their experiences with electrical stimulation of pain inhibition systems in chronic pain, whether directly on the nerve bundles (at the level of the first afferent sensory neuron), at the posterior horn of the spinal cord or at the deep cerebral level (sensitive thalamic and periaqueductal nuclei).

Techniques

Electrical neurostimulation can be done at four different sites which are, from the periphery to the centre, the skin, the sensory peripheral nerves, dorsal columns and the sensory thalamic nuclei (Fig. 4). Only the last three sites require surgery and implantation of a neurostimulator. The easiest and safest stimulation sites should be tried first. The aim is to provoke or stimulate "comfortable" electrical paraesthesia involving as much of the painful territory as possible.

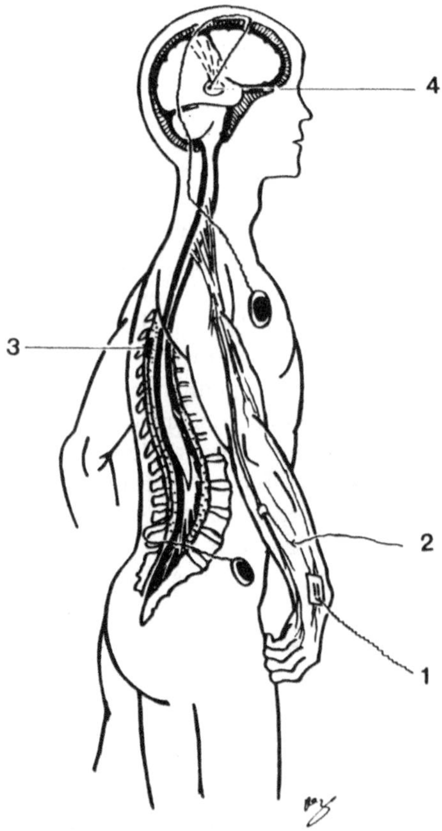

Fig. 4. Sites of analgesic techniques of electrical neurostimulation: *1* transcutaneous stimulation; *2* stimulation of peripheral nerves; *3* stimulation of spinal dorsal columns; *4* thalamic stimulation

Implantable Analgesic Neurostimulators (Fig. 5)

Arising directly from the technological experience with cardiac pacemakers, the neurostimulators [5, 13] are divided into two groups:

1. *Radiofrequency stimulators* have externally generated impulses. The implantable part is composed of an electrical stimulating electrode of which the active cathode is in contact with the nervous site and connected by a wire to a radiofrequency receptor. The electrodes differ according to the site of stimulation and the implantation technique used (directly with open surgery or percutaneously with stereotaxy).

An external part comprises a radiofrequency transmitter which allows for modulation and relay of the signal by an antenna placed on the skin. The most recent models incorporate several channels, allowing one to individually activate various electrode contacts.

2. *Totally implantable stimulators* have an implantable battery as the energy source. Battery life varies with stimulation strength and frequency, but is in the order of 5 years. These are more comfortable for the patient and can be turned on or off, activated by a magnet. They are programmed with the aid of a programming console allowing for individual variation as treatment evolves.

Fig. 5. Multiprogrammable implantable neurostimulators: *A* radiofrequency receiver; *B* totally implantable stimulator. With each stimulator is shown a four-contact electrode, implantable by laminectomy or by the percutaneous technique

Implantation Techniques

The implantation of the active cathode depends on the stimulation target [5, 13].

- For the stimulation of peripheral nerves, the ring-shaped cathode is directly implanted by open surgery on the peripheral nerve innervating the painful territory, for example the cubital or the sciatic nerve. In certain cases it can be percutaneously implanted, e.g. the trigeminal nerve.
- In spinal cord stimulation the unipolar, bipolar or quadripolar electrode is implanted in the epidural space adjacent to the dorsal columns (Fig. 6). The percutaneous procedure is non-invasive and can be carried out under local anaesthesia but allows perioperative verification of the site with the inherent risk of electrode displacement. In deep cerebral stimulation, electrode implantation requires specialised stereotactic techniques.

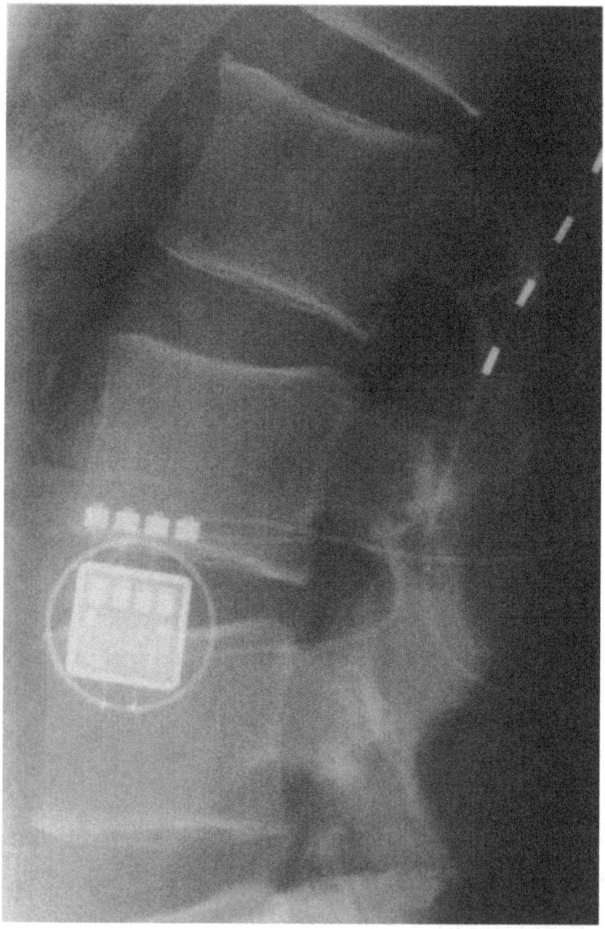

Fig. 6. Control radiograph of an implantable radiofrequency neurostimulator and its four-contact electrode

Stimulation Parameters

Regardless of the site of stimulation, peripheral or central, the aim is to provoke, by stimulation of sensory pathways (large myelinated fibres), electrical paresthesia over the complete pain territory. The topography of this paresthesia depends on correct and precise electrode placement. The stimulation parameters are specific and allow one to selectively activate the large myelinated fibres. Biphasic, symmetric and variable stimuli provoke a "comfortable, paraesthetic sensation". For this, one adjusts three variables: intensity, between 0 and 12 V, stimulation frequency, between 10 and 100 cycles/s and wavelength, 0.1 and 1 m/s. The stimulus is usually repeated at 10- or 20-min intervals three or four times a day. The duration of analgesia varies from one patient to the next, the stimulus being individually adapted as required.

Indications

The principle of analgesia by electrical neurostimulation is explained by the partial deafferentation in chronic secondary neurogenic pain. The pain is due to a modification of the somatotopic aesthesia in myelinated fibre injury. The most suitable indications are:
- Incomplete post-traumatic peripheral nerve or root lesions
- Partial brachial plexus lesions
- Amputation pain (phantom pain, stump pain, neuroma)
- Algodystrophic syndrome
- Incomplete paraplegic pain
- Most suitably of all, arachnoid plexus fibrosis, especially lumbar

The pain syndromes accompanying complete deafferentation constitute "painful anaesthesia" syndromes responding partially to neurostimulation and, in this case, only deep cerebral stimulation affords lasting analgesia. Intense pain due to nociceptive excess, such as cancer pain, is not ameliorated by this technique and is indeed a contraindication.

Even where there is a preferential indication, long-standing neurostimulation should only be undertaken after sufficiently long lasting percutaneous test stimulations have yielded beneficial results [5, 13].

Local, Spinal or Intraventricular Morphine Therapy

Neurophysiological Basis and Principles

Since 1975, numerous neurobiological experiments and clinical developments in spinal and central morphine action have given rise to local morphine therapy. The developments [2, 9] include:
- The discovery of opioid receptors in the CNS, especially in the spinal cord.

- In the spinal "animal", the selected inhibitory effect on nociceptive stimuli by the converging neurons in the gelatinous substance after intravenous or micro-ioncophoretically administered morphine.
- The demonstration that morphine administered directly into the cerebrospinal fluid (CSF) at the lumbar region in the rat and primate provoked a caudal analgesia which was intense and prolonged, implying the presence of opioid receptors, the effects being dose-dependent, stereospecific and reversible with naloxone.

In 1977, Wang [21] reported intense, selective and durable analgesia in patients with intractable pain following direct intrathecal injection of small doses of morphine (0.5–3.0 mg). The effect of this study was considerable with regard to both the development of the theory and subsequent therapies. Modes of administration are shown in Fig. 7.

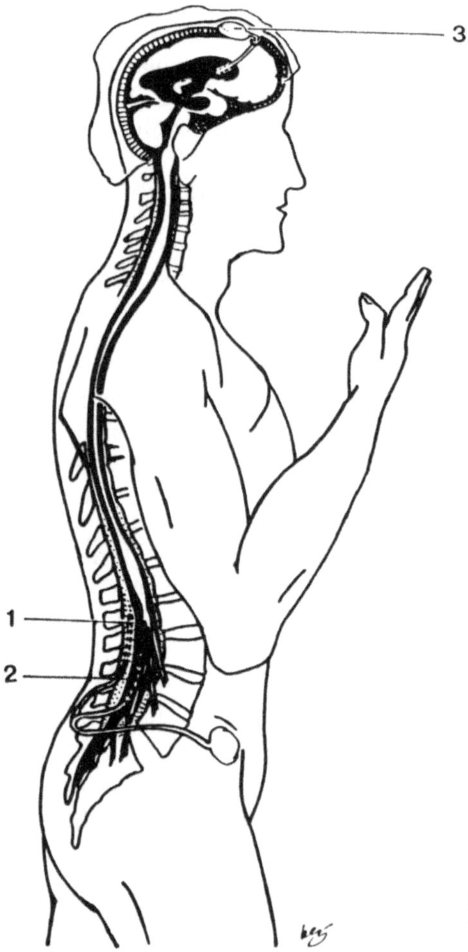

Fig. 7. Sites of surgical opioid administration: *1* lumbar epidural; *2* lumbar intrathecal; *3* intraventricular

The rapid development of this effective, mildly invasive, conservative and totally reversible method of chronic pain relief has been predominantly concerned with pain of malignant origin.

Techniques

Implantable Systems (Fig. 8)

Implantable systems are divided into two types:

1. *Access ports* require small reservoirs (0.5–2 ml) composed of external subcutaneously placed membranes permitting repeated percutaneous puncture. Their aim is to transform a lumbar puncture into an easy cutaneous injection. The different subsystems are made of biocompatible material. Their use necessitates repeated punture until an effective dose is reached. It is necessary to take rigorous aseptic precautions to prevent infectious complications, local sepsis or meningitis.
2. *Implantable pumps* bear the advantage that, having a reservoir, they allow the patient to enjoy some degree of autonomy. They are classified by their energy sources into chemical (gas, compression, fluorocarbon), mechanical and electrical. The pumps with gas propulsion have continuous flow (Infusaid). Their use is limited by not having an emergency stop in the event of overdosage, and to modify the dosage it is necessary to change the morphine concentration. The mechanical and electrical systems, however, allow one to programme various dosages (repeated bolus injection, continuous flow, on-demand facility etc.). However, the cost of these systems limits their use in the main to those patients with a limited life expectancy.

Mechanically activated transcutaneous pumps allow the repeated administration of 0.1 ml of solution. These systems, of acceptable cost, represent a compromise between simple, undertunnelled access ports and more sophisticated implantable pumps.

Implantation is carried out under either simple local or, preferably, neuroleptic anaesthesia.

Spinal implantation: The catheter is implanted with a Tuohy needle under fluoroscopic control by puncturing the intervertebral space L3–4 or L4–5. The distal end of the catheter is advanced to the intervertebral space T12–L1 (Fig. 7 and 9). The proximal end is connected to an implantable subcutaneous dosing device in either the abdominal thoracic or the external iliac space.

Long-term intraventricular implantation: This is achieved by implantation of an intraventricular catheter in the frontal horn or the right lateral ventricle, close to the foramen of Monro, accessed through a bore hole at the coronal suture approximately 3–4 cm from the median cranial line (Fig. 7 and 10).

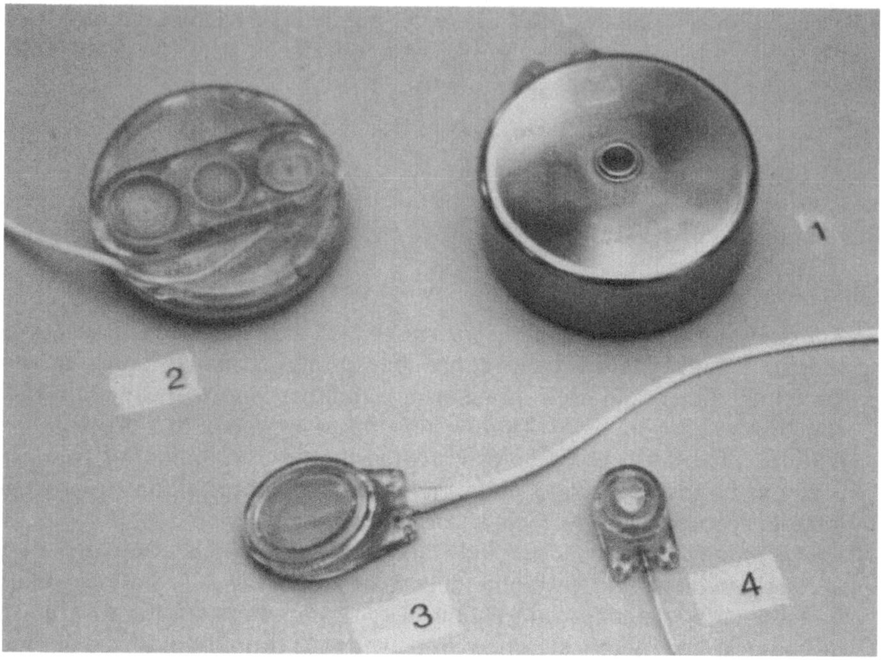

Fig. 8. Spinal port systems for opioid administration: *1* programmable pump (Synchromed Medtronic); *2* implantable mechanical pump (Secor Cordis); *3* standard spinal port; *4* miniaturized spinal port

This catheter is connected to a subcutaneous device in the skull or at some distance in the subclavicular space.

Morphine Solution

At the spinal level, we administer hyperbaric solutions (dextrose 7%) at a concentration of 5 mg morphine/ml. The use of a morphine solution "weighted" with glucose permits limitation of supraspinal perfusion of morphine, which carries the inherent risk of central respiratory depression. One can also observe, by pharmacokinetic studies in the CSF and plasma, the slower diffusion of morphine in hyperbaric solution than in normobaric solution. This gives longer-lasting analgesia and improves stability, glucose acting as a preservative.

Indications

The indications for local morphine therapy are based on rigorous clinical criteria:

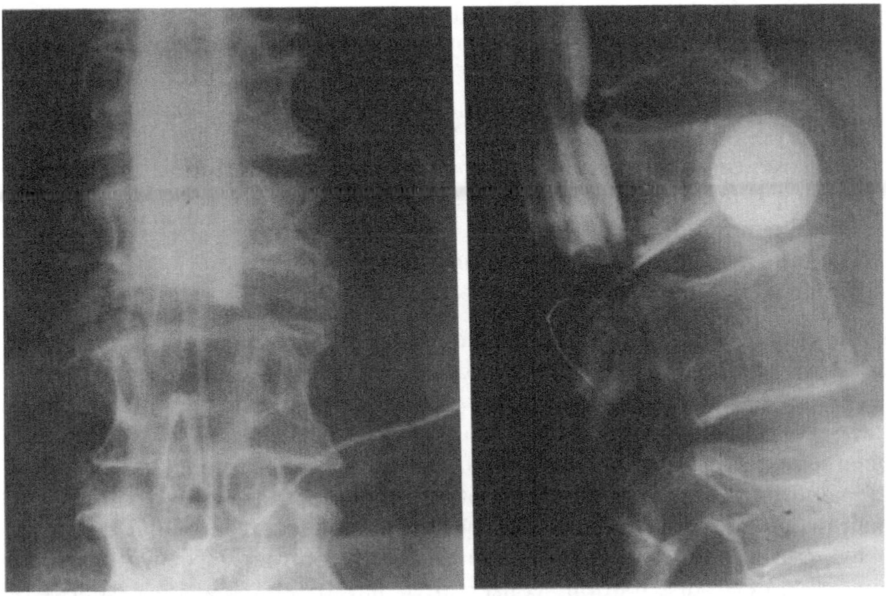

Fig. 9. Control radiographs of a port implanted at the lumbar level after opacification of the port and after opacification of the subarachnoid space

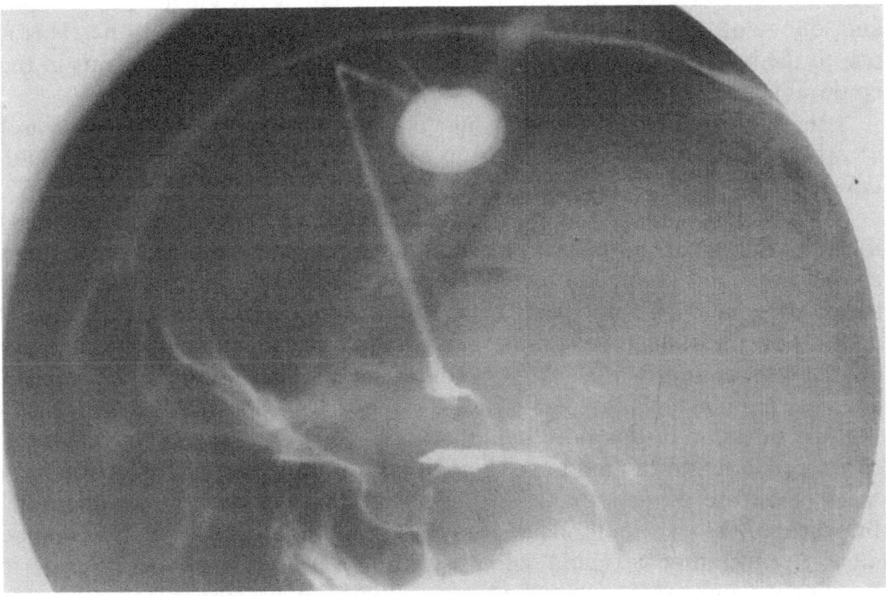

Fig. 10. Opacification of a port for intracerebroventricular opioid administration. The tip of the catheter is in the third ventricle

- Chronic refractory pain of neoplastic origin
- Refractory pain not ameliorated by medical therapy, especially systemic and oral opioids
- Bilateral, median or diffuse pain, that is to say pain not amenable to surgical percutaneous analgesic techniques
- The absence of general risks or complications such as intracranial hypertension, skin infections or general sepsis.
- The likelihood of benefit accruing from such therapy
- The informed consent of patient and family
- Circumstances favourable to subsequent treatment

If the origin of the pain is thoracic or subdiaphragmatic, suitability is confirmed by test administration of low-dose intrathecal morphine at the lumbar region (1–2.5 mg) to evaluate efficacy. A percutaneous catheter is placed in the subarachnoid space at the level of T12–L1 adjacent to the lumbar enlargement of the spinal cord. One can tunnel it subcutaneously to allow repeated injection of morphine or other opioids. On the other hand, if the pain is cephalic or diffuse, one can perform direct intraventricular injection.

Numerous publications have confirmed the efficacy, specificity, caudal and metameric distribution, conservative nature and low invasiveness of direct spinal low-dose morphine injection in the treatment of pain due to cancer. The observed results correlate perfectly with experimental data. After injection of low-dose morphine solution (1–2.5 mg), profound analgesia, predominantly of the lower limbs, follows after a latency period of 5–10 min and lasts 24–72 h. To provoke similar analgesia using epidural techniques, larger doses (5 mg) are required, the latency is longer (15–20 min) and, above all, the duration of analgesia is much shorter (12–24 h). This is due to the semi-systemic method of administration; veins are presents in the epidural space.

After low-dose intraventricular injection of morphine (1–2 mg) the onset of analgesia is equally rapid (5–10 min) and duration is even greater (1–8 days).

The analgesic efficacy and low incidence of side effects after low-dose intrathecal lumbar or intraventricular injection of morphine ensures this conservative and reversible technique a place in the treatment of refractory neoplastic pain. The perspective of this technique gives hope of clinical application for other types of pain, especially of benign origin, and depends on the use of more efficacious opioids and the development of suitably adapted implantable devices. Our experience brings us to the conclusion that the injection of low-dose hyperbaric morphine is indicated in refractory chronic pain limited to the lower limbs. After failure of spinal injection or in cases of diffuse thoracic pain, intraventricular administration is preferable. In practice, the two methods of local morphine administration are complementary. Intrathecal opioid administration represents a new concept in functional neurosurgery: “local pharmacological neurosurgery”.

Surgical Strategies

The objects of surgical treatment in chronic pain are threefold:
Efficacy: immediate and durable analgesia
Safety: the surgical intervention must be the least traumatic possible and the patient's general health status should be unchanged
Acceptable cost: with regard to the technique as well as the socio-professional consequences for the patient during follow-up

Patient Selection Criteria

The most effective pain of treatment is suppression of the cause. Before considering surgical intervention for chronic refractory pain, the cause should be rigorously investigated and proven organic, that is to say, it should not persist after reversal of mechanical nerve compression. This fundamental principle is well illustrated by the refractory sciatic pain secondary to lumbar disc surgery. The progress made in scanning techniques has shown that in some cases refractory pain of this type is due to radicular compression by residual disc sequestra.

Prior to proposing surgical treatment, one should ensure that the pain cannot be effectively controlled by conservative medical therapy. Often it is only necessary to reconsider systemic analgesic therapy, using new medications and combinations. In the same way, the ineffectiveness of other conservative therapies such as transcutaneous stimulation, acupuncture and physiotherapy must be verified.

Psychological evaluation of the patient is a very important step. Sometimes a simple conversation will suffice, in other cases one must combine psychometric tests with investigations into the origin of the pain to eliminate contraindications to surgery. Patients who have already been operated upon may have iatrogenically modified sensitivity to pain. The sensory disturbances are intrinsically related to the initial pathology, and one may therefore be obliged to modify classical neurosurgical indications, for example, in the case of essential trigeminal neuralgia following extended desensitisation by neurolysis (alcohol, neurotomy, thermocoagulation). The neurophysiological evaluation of refractory pain syndrome should always be rigorous.

It is important to ascertain the following when selecting neurosurgical techniques:

- The topographic extent of the pain
- Whether focal localised truncal pain is monoradicular or polyradicular.
- Whether other nonsystemic pain is regional or diffuse.

Modification of pain sensitivity, by comparing with other cutaneous areas, particularly the contralateral dermatome. A classical clinical pin-prick or light-touch test is complemented by quantitative measurement.

- Whether the triggering point of the electrical peripheral nerve, e.g. the saphenous nerve, is coupled with the reflex threshold (EMG of ischio-

femoral muscles). This allows quantification of analgesia and is repeatable and of comparative value.
- The benign or malignant aetiology of the pain.
- The patient's life expectancy.
- Concomitant risk factors.

Finally, it is often useful to complete investigations with percutaneous tests to assess the possible outcome of neurosurgical intervention; for instance, transitory nerve blockade by long-acting anaesthestic solutions before performing definitive neurolysis. This is also the principle behind prolonged percutaneous epidural stimulation before deciding to implant a spinal cord stimulator and lumbar intrathecal administration of morphine before implanting a port system.

Choice of Surgical Technique

The choice of surgical technique is dictated not only by the site and extent of pain but also by the aetiology and degree of associated sensory nerve injury. It follows, therefore, that in pain of benign origin the technique indicated depends essentially on the sensitivity of the tissues in the painful region and that excess nociceptive stimulation must oppose the neurogenic pain provoked by deafferentation and accompanying hypoaesthesia or complete anaesthesia. This is well illustrated by facial pain of trigeminal origin: usually, the essential trigeminal neuralgia does not follow directly from the actual facial injury; but is due to excessive nociception. In this neuralgia, evolving from recurring crises and seen predominantly in old people, the usual technique is percutaneous selective thermocoagulation of the trigeminal ganglion. However, the thermal neurolysis is ineffective unless accompanied by anaesthesia to hard and occasionally light touch, limited to the area of pain insensibility. This localised sensory deprivation is generally well accepted by the patient; however, it is dangerous when it involves the ophthalmic territory, as corneal anaesthesia predisposes to the development of corneal ulcers. Therefore, when facial neuralgia involves the ophthalmic territory, especially in a young subject, it is logical to propose an open surgical technique, for example microvascular decompression.

On the other hand, in the rare cases of trigeminal neuralgia that continuously evolve accompanied by sensory problems (neuropathy of traumatic iatrogenic origin) it is useless and also dangerous to aggravate the symptoms by performing percutaneous neurolysis. Alternative therapy includes electrical neurostimulation, initally transcutaneous and then, in the case of failure, of the trigeminal ganglion.

In the same way, analgesic neurostimulation is indicated in all other neurogenic pain of benign origin accompanied by sensory disafferentiation; this includes incomplete peripheral nerve lesions, arachnoid inflammations and pain in paraplegia or amputation. The choice of technique of electrical stimulation progresses from peripheral transcutaneous stimulation to central thalamic medullary stimulation.

In severe nociceptive pain of neoplastic origin, options have been greatly simplified since the development of local morphine therapy. This low-dose, highly successful, easily performed percutaneous procedure may also be used in pain due to excess nociception provoked by invasion of nervous plexuses. Apart from the rare unilateral and localised cancer pain syndromes meriting percutaneous surgical section (radicotomy or more often, cervical cordotomy), for example pain due to limb sarcomas, the majority of pain is bilateral, median and/or diffuse. In these cases, the site of local morphine administration depends on the area of pain; lumbar peridural for lower body pain, intraventricular for diffuse or upper body pain. Today, there is only a limited place for disruptive surgery in the therapy of neoplastic pain, and its relative efficacy does not justify the risk of complications, especially the creation of new pain due to disafferentiation.

Conclusions

The large number of surgical techniques proposed to treat chronic refractory pain reflect the complexity of the subject. Irreducible pain is multifactorial in origin and there is no one universal solution. Beginning with initial rigorous evaluation, the choice of treatment depends on adherence to certain general rules, and the surgical strategy selected should be the least traumatic of those that would be effective. To achieve this goal one must:

- Have a large technical repertoire, a multidisciplinary approach and experienced personnel
- Use and eliminate all possible conservative techniques before considering destructive techniques
- Give priority to percutaneous methods over open surgery
- Choose peripheral targets before acting at the centre

Recent work on neurophysiological, electrical and chemical pain control mechanisms allows one to fulfil these requirements. In 1940, René Leriche, the pioneer of "pain surgery" introduced, as well as his hypotheses on the role of the sympathetic nervous system, the idea of functional surgery based on the physiology of pain: "Instead of crudely interrupting the sensory pathways we should act with their functions in mind, using the experience and methods of this physiologically based surgery that has been developed over the past 15 years".

Acknowledgements. I would like to express my gratitude to Dr. Jacques Richaud, neurosurgeon, and to Monsieur Francois Caraoue, laboratory technician for the illustrations. This chapter was translated from the original French text by Dr. Jean Paul Meisch, Department of Anaesthesiology, University of Heidelberg, FRG.

References

1. Behar M, Olshwano D, Magora F, Davidson JT (1979) Epidural morphine in treatment of pain. Lancet i:572–578
2. Besson JM, Lazorthes Y (1984) Sustance opioïdes médullaires et analgésie. Aspects fondamentaux et applications cliniques. INSERM, Paris, 127:1–500
3. Dandy WE (1925) Section of the sensory roots of the trigeminal nerve at the pons. Preliminary report and operative procedure. J Hop Hosp Bull 36:105
4. Guillaume J, de Seze S, Mazars G (1949) Chirurgie érébro-spinale de la douieur. Presses universitaires de France, Paris
5. Lazorthes Y, Upton ARM (1985) Neurostimulation: an overview. Future Publishing Company, New York
6. Lazorthes Y, Verdie JC (1978) Traitement des douleurs irréductibles. Les techniques antigésiques percutanées. Pierre Fabre, Castres
7. Lazorthes Y, Verdie JC (1979) Radiofrequency coagulation of the petrous ganglion in glossopharyngeal neuralgia. Neurosurg 4:12–16
8. Lazorthes Y, Verdie JC, Lagarrigue J (1976) Thermocoagulation percutanée des neris rachidiens à visée analgcaique. Neurochir 22:445–453
9. Lazorthes Y, Gouarmeres C, Verdie JC, Montsarrat B, Bastede R, Campan L et al (1980) Analgésie par injection intrathernie de morphine. Etude pharmacosinétique et applications aux douleurs irréductibles. Neurochir 26A:159–164
10. Lazorthes Y, Verdie JC, Bastide R, Lavados A, Descouens D (1985) Spinal versus for cancer pain. Appl Neurophysiol 48:234–241
11. Leriche R (1940) La chirurgie de la douleur. Masson, Paris
12. Rosomoff ML, Caroll F, Brown J. Sheptak P (1965) Percutaneous radiofrequency cervical cordotomy. Techn J Neurosurg 23:639–644
13. Sedan R, Lazorthes Y (1978) La stimulation électrique thérapeutique. Neurochir 24:1–138
14. Shealy CM, Mortimer JT, Reswick J (1967) Electrical inhibition of pain by stimulation of the dorsal column : preliminary clinical reports. Anesth Analg 46:489–494
15. Sindou M (1972) Etude de la jonction radiculo-médullaire postérieure. La radicellotomie postérieure sélective dans la chirurgie de la douleur. Thèse Méd Lyon
16. Spiller WG, Martin E (1912) The treatment of pain of organic origin in the lower part of the body by division of the anterolateral column of the spinal cord. JAMA 58:1489–1490
17. Sweet WH, Wepsic JQ (1968) treatment of chronic pain by stimulation of fibers or primary afferent neurons. Trans Am Neurol Assoc 93:103–105
18. Sweet WH, Wepsic JG (1974) Controlled the mocoagulation of trigeminal ganglion and rootlets for differential destruction of pain fibers. I : Trigeminal neuralgia. J Neurosurg 35:143
19. Talairach J, Szikla G, Tournoux P, Bonn P, Bancaud J (1962) Le chirurgie stéréotaxique hypophysaire. Confia Neurol, Basel 22:204–213
20. White JC, Sweet WH (1969) Pain and the neurosurgeon. A 40 years experience. Thomas, Springfield
21. Wang JK (1979) Analgesic effets of intrathecally administred morphine. Reg Anesthesia 4:2–3
22. Yaksh TL (1978) Analgesic actions of intrathecal opiates in cat and primate. Brain Res 153:205–210

Interpleural Pain Treatment

PER H. ROSENBERG

Interpleural regional analgesia was introduced for postoperative pain relief after cholecystectomy, breast surgery and renal surgery [1]. This analgesic method has since been applied in the treatment of post-thoracotomy pain [2–4], pain from multiple rib fractures [5], postherpetic neuralgia [6] and pain due to chronic pancreatitis [7] or pancreatic cancer [8]. Long-term analgesia in a few patients with pain from lung cancer with metastases has been achieved with interpleural bupivacaine [9, 10].

Mechanisms of Action

The position of the patient may affect the distribution of the interpleurally administered local anaesthetic to a major extent [11, 12]. The cranio-caudal distribution of contrast medium-containing bupivacaine solution (30 ml) was between the levels T3 and L1 when the patient was supine and between T5 and L1 in the lateral position [12]. The positional dependence of the primary distribution of an interpleurally injected local anaesthetic solution may in part explain the variable analgesic results obtained in post-thoracotomy pain control.

Generally, the analgesic effect appears to be better after surgery in the upper splanchnic region than after thoracotomy. This suggests an important involvement of splanchnic nerve block in the mechanism of action of interpleural regional analgesia.

Intercostal Nerve Block

The intercostal nerve roots are least protected at the costovertebral angle, at which site they are covered only by the pleura and the posterior intercostal fascia. Transpleural penetration of local anaesthetics is rapid and concentration-dependent [13]. With the patient in the supine position there is marked collection of local anaesthetic solution posterior and more on the mediastinal side of the interpleural space [12]. Subjective and objective analgesia via intercostal nerve block has been reported in patients with multiple rib fractures [5] and after cholecystectomy or renal surgery [14] during interpleural bupivacaine treatment.

Sympathetic Blockade

The main portion of the thoracic sympathetic chain is separated from the pleural cavity only by the parietal pleura. The reported development of Horner's syndrome when the head end of the table was tilted down [7, 15], suggests a significant involvement of the blockade of the sympathetic nervous system in interpleural regional analgesia.

The major and minor splanchnic nerves derive from the 6th–9th and the 10th–11th thoracic sympathetic ganglia, respectively. The favourable effect of interpleural regional analgesia on upper abdominal visceral pain, both acute and chronic, is probably due to blockade of the splanchnic nerves at the thoracic level.

Pleural Analgesia

The parietal pleura, particularly in the costal portion, has a rich sensory nerve supply derived both from the intercostal nerves and the phrenic nerve. Therefore, topical pleural analgesia is probably one of the components of interpleural regional analgesia.

Phrenic Nerve Block

There is no clinical evidence that the phrenic nerve trunk itself would be blocked to the degree that diaphragmatic motion would become impaired. Postoperatively, significant improvement of the respiratory function has been reported [16] during interpleural regional analgesia after cholecystectomy, with no diaphragmatic paralysis.

Toxicological Aspects of Interpleural Analgesia

In the survey by Strømskag et al. [17], occasional toxic reactions caused by large doses of either bupivacine or lidocaine are reported. The authors, who undoubtedly have great experience of the interpleural technique, conclude that a dose of up to 20 ml 0.5% bupivacaine in adults is safe.

A reason for the lack of toxic reactions, as well as for occasional relatively poor analgesia in post-thoracotomy patients [2, 4], may be the loss of a significant amount of the interpleurally instilled dose of local anaesthetic via the chest drains.

Interpleural Analgesia for Cancer Pain

There are only a few case reports [8–10] and no controlled studies on the efficacy of interpleural regional analgesia in the control of cancer pain.

Surprisingly, long-lasting pain relief has been obtained in patients with pancreatic cancer as well as in chronic pancreatitis; in a cancer patient 8 ml 0.5% bupivacaine injected twice at 24-h-interval caused complete pain relief for 12 h each time, and the patient could be managed without opioid medication for at least 3 months thereafter [8]. Interestingly, interpleural instillation of phenol had been under consideration in this particular patient.

Patients with lung cancer and chest wall metastases have obtained good pain relief for several weeks when 40 mg of methylprednisolone acetate was added to the interpleural bupivacaine solution [10]. Another patient with lung cancer pain was managed by interpleural injection of 10 ml 0.25% bupivacaine one to four times daily for 7 weeks [9].

Complications

Strømskag et al. [17] have recently published a report on side effects and complications related to interpleural analgesia. The most common complication is pneumothorax (2%). In one study [16] mild cases of pneumothorax occurred in 19%. Occasional cases of pleural effusion, bacterial infection, puncture of the lung, catheter rupture, Horner's syndrome and systemic local anaesthetic toxicity have been reported [17].

Conclusion

Interpleural analgesia in cancer pain is an alternative, but certainly not the first choice in any patient. In patients after thoracotomy for lung cancer and in whom postoperative pain relief has been achieved with the interpleural technique, analgesic therapy can obviously be continued via the interpleural catheter. Due to decreased immunocompetence in such patients, the risk of infection is enhanced.

The interesting and promising results presented by Klein and Klein [10] should probably be pursued further. Controlled studies comparing interpleural analgesia by local anaesthetic plus methylprednisolone with e.g. epidural analgesia in the control of lung cancer pain should be performed. There is also a need for controlled studies on the usefulness of the interpleural technique in pancreatic cancer pain.

The use of interpleural neurolysis (phenol) must be further evaluated in careful animal experiments before any therapeutic attempts are made in patients.

References

1. Reiestad F, Strømskag KE (1986) Intrapleural catheter in the management of postoperative pain. Reg Anaesth 11:89–91
2. Rosenberg PH, Scheinin BM-A, Lepänatalo MJA, Lindfors O (1987) Continuous interpleural infusion of bupivacaine for analgesia after thoracotomy. Anesthesiology 67:811–813

3. McIlvane WB, Knox RF, Fennessey PV, Goldstein M (1988) Continuous infusion of bupivacaine via interpleural catheter for analgesia after thoracotomy in children. Anesthesiology 69:261–264
4. Symreng T, Gomez MN, Rossi N (1989) Intrapleural bupivacaine v. saline after thoracotomy – effects on pain and lung function – a double-blind study. J Cardiothorac Anesth 3:144–149
5. Rocco A, Reiestad F, Gudman J, McKay W (1987) Intrapleural administration of local anesthetics for pain relief in patients with multiple rib fractures. A preliminary report. Reg Anaesth 12:10–14
6. Sihota MK, Holmblad BR (1988) Horner's syndrome after interpleural anesthesia with bupivacaine for postherpetic neuralgia. Acta Anaesthesiol Scand 32:593–594
7. Sihota MK, Holmblad BR, Ikuta PT, Candido KD (1988) Successful pain management of chronic pancreatitis with interpleural technique. Reg Anaesth 13:S33
8. Durrani Z, Winnie AP, Ikuta P (1988) Interpleural catheter analgesia for pancreatic pain. Anesth Analg 67:479–481
9. Fineman SP (1989) Long-term post-thoracotomy cancer pain management with interpleural bupivacaine. Anesthesiology 68:694–697
10. Klein DS, Klein PW (1991) Intermittent interpleural injection of bupivacaine and methylprednisolone for analgesia in metastatic thoracic neoplasm. Clin J Pain 7:232–236
11. Riegler FX, Pelligrino DA, VadeBoncouer TR (1988) An animal model of intrapleural analgesia. Anesthesiology 69:A365
12. Strømskag KE, Hauge O, Steen PA (1990) Distribution of local anesthetics injected into the interpleural space, studied by computerized tomography. Acta Anaesthesiol Scand 34:323–326
13. Turner D, Williams S, Heavner J (1989) Pleural permeability to local anesthetics – the influence of concentration, pH, and local anesthetic combinations. Reg Anaesth 14:128–132
14. Van Kleef JW, Burm AGL, Vletter AA (1990) Single-dose interpleural versus intercostal blockade: nerve block characteristics and plasma concentration profiles after administration of 0.5% bupivacaine with epinephrine. Anesth Analg 70:484–488
15. Parkinson SK, Mueller JB, Rich TJ, Little WL (1989) Horner's syndrome associated with interpleural catheter injection of local anesthetic. Anesth Analg 68:61–62
16. Brismar B, Pettersson N, Tokics L, Strandberg A, Hedenstierna G (1987) Postoperative analgesia with intrapleural administration of bupivacaine-adrenaline. Acta Anaesthesiol Scand 31:515–520
17. Strømskag KE, Minor B, Steen PA (1990) Side effects and complications related to interpleural analgesia: an update. Acta Anaesthesiol Scand 34:473–477

Percutaneous Dorsal Root Ganglia Lesions for Cancer Pain

David Niv

Intractable pain of malignant origin is sometimes limited to 1–3 dermatomes. Patients suffering from such pain are capable of indicating the area of maximum discomfort, and in most cases, pressure applied directly to that area intensifies the pain. In our experience, patients with localized pain generally demand a localized solution for their pain. In contrast to patients experiencing pain in diffused sites, those with localized pain agree to receive opioid drugs only as a last resort and after exhausting all known localized therapies.

Uematsu et al. [1] in 1974 were the first to describe a technique for percutaneous dorsal root ganglia lesioning by radiofrequency for the relief of localized intractable pain. The procedure consists of inserting a needle which is isolated except for its tip, localizing the dorsal root ganglia in question under X-ray and with the aid of electrical stimulation, and then performing a radiofrequency lesion in its sensory component. The technique can be easily learned by anesthesiologists skilled in regional anesthesia, but it is no less important to understand the indications for selecting the candidates and performing the procedure within the framework of a multidisciplinary cancer pain approach. The following case report presents an example of a patient managed with this procedure:

A 56-year-old female suffered sharp localized pain in the left side of her abdomen. The dermatomal distribution of her pain was L1. Two years earlier she underwent a total abdominal hysterectomy because of carcinoma of her uterus. No examination pain could be evoked on direct local pressure. The differential diagnosis was between iliac crest metastasis, referred pain from abdominal recurrence of the tumor, and spinal metastasis. Whole body bone scan revealed iliac crest metastasis. However the diagnosis of the level of pain distribution was confirmed only by a paravertebral block of the left L1 nerve root with 2 ml 1.5% lidocaine. Subsequently percutaneous radiofrequency lesions of T12, L1 and L2 left ganglia were performed in one session, obtaining good pain relief for 12 months of follow-up.

Patients and Methods

Patients with evidence of malignancy in the periphery and localized pain limited to one or two adjacent dermatomes have to be assessed for their suitability for the procedure. The pain intensity under consideration should be severe and not controlled with mild to moderate analgesics. Additional suitable patients are those who have tried opioid analgesics but found them to have adverse effects or interfere with their quality of life.

It is important to perform an X-ray-guided paravertebral nerve block with local anesthetic (2 ml) in order to ascertain the nociceptive pathway, determine the patient's reaction to pain relief, and also to afford him the opportunity to experience the referred numbness that often follows a destructive procedure and thus help him to decide whether or not to have it done. Pain relief exceeding the expected duration of the local anesthetic effect represents an additional diagnostic prediction for the success of the procedure.

The technique used is based on that described by Uematsu et al. [1] and later by Sluiter and Mehta [2]. The patient is positioned prone on a radiolucent operating table with mild flexion of the spine. With the aid of a C-arm radiographic image intensifier, the level of the procedure can be verified and the skin infiltrated with local anesthetic 5–8 cm laterally to the spinal process, depending on whether it is performed in the cervical, thoracic, or lumbar region, and 1–2 cm caudal to the intervertebral foramen in question. Subsequently a radiofrequency 22 G needle probe is inserted in an anterolateral and slightly cranial direction until contact is made with the transverse process of the vertebra involved. The needle should then be walked in a more anterior and caudal direction until it slips into the foramen. The correct position of the needle's tip should be exactly in line with the facet joint spaces on the anteroposterior projection of the image intensifier, and in the posterior part of the foramen on the lateral projection.

Verification of the needle's position has to be obtained also by a series of electrical stimuli at a frequencies of 5 and 100 Hz for motor and sensory response respectively. The ideal placement is where sensory response in the painful dermatome can be elicited with stimuli below 0.5 V intensity and motor response not below twice the sensory threshold.

After establishing the site for the lesion, 1 ml 2% lidocaine should be injected through the needle. The thermal lesion is regulated to 70° C and held for 90 s. Before the needle is finally withdrawn 40 mg of methylprednisolone are injected.

Results

The clinical data and outcome results of 50 patients treated by the procedure in the last 3 years are summarized in Table 1.

The mean age of the patients was 62.5 years (range 43–71). The total number of lesions was 110 (mean 2.2 lesions per patient). The period of time which elapsed to establish the outcome was 3 months. Thirty-one patients (62%) had good results – virtually pain-free and requiring analgesics only occasionally. Fourteen patients (28%) had fair relief requiring reduced doses of moderate analgesics. Five patients (10%) had no reduction of their

Table 1. Clinical data and results 3 months after dorsal root ganglia lesioning

No. of patients	M/F	Primary carcinoma	Main location of pain	Results Nil	Fair	Good
12	9/ 3	Melanoma	Legs, abdomen		2	10
8	–/ 8	Genitalia	Pelvis, abdomen	2	3	3
7	–/ 7	Breast	Chest, ribs		2	5
5	5/ –	Prostate	Pelvis, abdomen	1	2	2
5	4/ 1	Bronchia and mediastinum	Chest, ribs		2	3
4	2/ 2	Alimentary tract	Abdomen, hip	1	1	2
4	2/ 2	Lymphoma	Hip, femur		1	3
2	2/ –	Leukemia	Hip		1	1
2	2/–	Bladder	Hip			2
1	–/ 1	Kidney	Low back	1		
50	26/24			5	14	31

Table 2. Side effects of 110 ganglia lesions

Side effect	No. of patients	Management	Duration
Neuralgic pain with hyperesthesia	11	Tricyclic anti-depressants	5–6 weeks
Hypoesthesia to pinprick	26	No treatment	1 month
Hypoalgesia	2	No treatment	9–11 months
Pneumothorax	1	Chest drainage	3 days
Occipital headache	1	Analgesics	2 days

pain, therefore requiring opioid analgesics to control it. Analysis of results 12 months after the procedure revealed that 48% of the patients still experienced a beneficial effect from the procedure, grading the pain relief in the related dermatomes as good. Eleven of the patients developed neuralgic pain with hyperesthesia in the distribution of the treated dermatome. This was noted 1 week after operation, managed with tricyclic anti-depressants, and lasted for 5–6 weeks (Table 2). Slight loss of sensation to pinprick was found in 26 of the patients within 2 weeks of the procedure. This hypoesthesia was no longer detectable after 1 month.

Two patients developed hypoalgesia which persisted for 9–11 months. No motor deficit developed in any patient, nor did any loss of control of movement. Patients were discharged to their homes 2 h following the procedure, except for two patients, one who developed pneumothorax following a thoracic procedure and a second who developed post-dural-puncture headache. The pneumothorax was treated with a drain and the patient was discharged from the hospital on the 3rd day after the procedure. The post-dural-headache resolved itself with analgesics only, and on the 2nd day the patient was sent home.

Discussion

Since Uematsu et al. first described the technique of percutaneous radiofrequency rhizotomy in 1974 [1], various authors have reported their experiences using this technique not only in cancer patients but also in patients with postherpetic neuralgia, postsurgical and posttraumatic pain, and for patients with "failed back" [2–5].

This method has many advantages, such as simplicity of procedure, minimal stay in hospital, and the possibility of assessing the results almost immediately. Other advantages of this technique versus open surgery of nerve roots include an awake, aware patient who is able to verbally respond and cooperate. The patient, while being electrode-stimulated, can be of help in localizing the nerve root responsible for the distribution of his pain. His reaction to the stimulation is important in determining the proximity of the electrode to the sensory part of the ganglion, and he can also assess the efficacy of the local anesthetic injected before making the lesion.

Letcher and Goldring [6] studied the effect of thermocoagulation of peripheral nerves and found that the small-diameter nerve fibers are the first to undergo damage as the heat rises. The idea of a selective lesion, i.e., maximal damage of nociceptive small myelinated and unmyelinated nerve fibers and minimal damage of the larger mechano- and proprioceptive fibers, is the target of the procedure. For this purpose most authors suggest a heat of 70°–80° C as ideal [2, 3, 5].

According to Smith et al. [7] small and large fibers are destroyed indiscriminately. In Dubuisson's view [4], thermocoagulation of large-diameter afferents as well contributes to the success of the procedure. In cancer, herpes zoster, and other conditions associated with deafferentation pain, stimulating afferents of large diameter by light touch or by brushing of hairs may evoke intense burning pain. It is therefore difficult to establish to what extent it is important to preserve the large-diameter afferents.

Major importance must be attributed to not lesioning the large motor efferent fibers. Anatomically the dorsal root ganglion is distinct from the motor nerve fibers, and therefore by serial electrical testing the tip of the electrode can be accurately placed in the ganglion. Furthermore, a lesion at the ganglion level involves not only the body cells of fibers travelling via the posterior horns of the cord, but also the body cells of sensory fibers which enter the cord via the anterior horns [8].

Recent studies have shown that the dorsal root ganglion undergoes modifications of its structure and activity following peripheral nerve damage [9,

10]. It is possible that the spontaneous discharges seen in the ganglia after peripheral damage contribute to the pain and that thermocoagulation of its structure reduces it. Moreover, lesions within the ganglion frame affect the ganglion cells, thus preventing regeneration of nerve fibers and the accompanying spontaneous burst of discharges as seen with peripheral nerve lesions and neuromas [11, 12].

It has been known for nearly a century [13, 14] that each dermatome is innervated by more than one nerve root. After establishing the area of maximum pain and the corresponding nerve root, we preferred in most of the cases to perform lesions on both adjacent ganglia as well. Although some reports argue the correlation between an effective root block and a good response to nerve section [15], we believe that blocks remain additional useful tools in ascertaining the segment involved. If, however, the pain fails to disappear after performing repeated blocks, application of a lesion will be of no value [15].

In summary, percutaneous radiofrequency lesioning of dorsal root ganglia is a very effective method if seen in the proper light. It is not the panacea for pain control in cancer patients, but in the framework of a multidisciplinary approach where many other methods are available, and when accurate selection of patients with localized pain is made, this technique can be very effective and reduce the amount of analgesics otherwise taken by the patient. The simplicity of the method and the low rate of side effects make it an additional tool for the control of localized cancer pain.

References

1. Uematsu S, Udvarhelyi GB, Benson DW, Siebens AA (1974) Percutaneous radiofrequency rhizotomy. Surg Neurol 2:319–325
2. Sluiter ME, Mehta M (1981) Treatment of chronic neck and back pain by percutaneous thermal lesions. In: Lipton S, Miles J (eds) Persistent pain. Modern methods of treatment, vol. 3. Academic, London, pp 141–179
3. Nash TP (1986) Percutaneous radiofrequency lesioning of dorsal root ganglia for intractable pain. Pain 24:67–73
4. Dubuisson D (1989) Root surgery. In: Wall PD, Melzack R (eds) Textbook of pain, 2nd edn. Churchill Livingstone, Edinburgh, pp 784–794
5. Sluiter ME (1988) The use of radiofrequency lesions for pain relief in failed back patients. Int Disabil Stud 10:37–43
6. Letcher FS, Goldring S (1968) The effect of radiofrequency current and heat on peripheral nerve action potential in the cat. J Neurosurg 29:42–47
7. Smith HP, McWhorter JM, Challa VR (1981) Radiofrequency neurolysis in a clinical model. Neuropathological correlation. J Neurosurg 55:246–253
8. Coggeshall RE, Applebaum MB, Frazen M, Stubbs TB, Sykes MT (1975) Unmyelinated axons in human ventral roots, a possible explanation for the failure of dorsal rhizotomy to relieve pain. Brain 98:157–166
9. Wall PD, Devor M (1983) Sensory afferent impulses originate from dorsal root ganglia as well as from the periphery in normal and nerve-injured rats. Pain 17:327–339
10. Burchiel K (1984) Effects of electrical and mechanical stimulation on two foci of spontaneous activity which develop in primary afferent neurons after peripheral axotomy. Pain 18:249–265

11. Wall P, Gutnick M (1974) Properties of afferent nerve impulses originating from a neuroma. Exp Neurol 43:580–593
12. Govrin-Lippman R, Devor M (1978) Ongoing activity in severed nerves: source and variation with time. Brain Res 159:406–410
13. Sherrington CS (1898) Experiments in the examination of the spinal nerves. II. Philos Trans Soc London [B] 190:45–186
14. Foerster O (1933) The dermatomes in man. Brain 56:1–39
15. Bonica JJ (1974) Floor discussion: dorsal rhizotomy. Adv Neurol 4:626

Peptides for Analgesia: Intrathecal Administration

RICHARD D. PENN

The possibility of using spinally active peptides for pain relief has become a practical reality with the development of catheter systems and pumps to chronically deliver these agents. In this article I will outline the progress we have made in using one such agent, octreotide, in cancer patients, and then consider the direction in which I think the field may develop.

Before discussing specific results, some principles of delivery of intrathecal medications need to be considered [8]. The most obvious advantage of the technique is that the blood-brain barrier is circumvented. This means that complex polar molecules which cannot penetrate the barrier can be used. Another equally important advantage of direct perfusion into the cerebral spinal fluid (CSF) is that a high concentration of drug can be placed near the receptor sites where it is bound. Rexed layers II and III of the spinal cord, where neurotransmitters modulate incoming sensory signals, are just a few millimeters away. Drugs placed in the CSF can slowly diffuse through the cord to these sites of action. If continuous delivery methods are employed using an external or implanted pump, a steady-state gradient will be created which drives the drug into the cord tissue. For polar, poorly lipid-soluble drugs, a gradient will be created not only from CSF to the tissue but also from the lumbar CSF to the cervical region. For example, after several hours of continuous infusion, morphine has a lumbar-to-cervical ratio of 5:1 [3]. Thus a specific regional delivery to the lower part of the spine is achieved, and central side effects will be reduced. If the drug is given by bolus instead of continuously, very high concentrations will result for short periods of time and CSF flow will carry the medicine up the neuraxis and could cause significant central side effects. Thus, the safest and most effective way to give analgesics spinally, be they narcotics, local anesthetics or peptides, is by slow perfusion.

The corollary to this point is that lipid-soluble or rapidly biodegradable compounds make poor candidates for slow infusion. They do not distribute over a large region nor will they be able to penetrate the spinal tissue deep enough to get to their receptor sites. As an example, midazolam, a lipid-soluble GABA agonist, has been infused by drug pump for spasticity [5]. No changes in spasticity occurred because of too rapid uptake of drug by superficial layers of the cord and loss across the arachnoid and dura into the systemic circulation. In fact, drowsiness resulted because the midazolam redistributed from the CSF to the systemic circulation and then to the brain. An example of peptide degradation is the use of somatostatin for pain. Although it is a polar compound and distributes well in the CSF, it is rapidly broken down in the neural tissue [7]. For that reason much higher doses have to be used than when a compound not degraded by neural enzymes is used. This is an important consideration when peptides and/or agonists are chosen for infusion. Since powerful degradation systems are found in the nervous system to limit the spread of neurotransmitters, naturally released peptides may be a poor choice for this mode of therapy.

The concept of using nonopiates intraspinally for pain has been the logical outgrowth of new knowledge about the converging circuits going to the dorsal horn neurons and the various neurotransmitters and modulators which exist in that region. The rationale for somatostatin use dates back to the observation that somatostatin is localized in intrinsic interneurons of the superficial region of the dorsal horn [9] and that it has an inhibitory effect [15]. More recent neurophysiological experiments by Sandkühler have elegantly demonstrated somatostatin's inhibition of nociceptive responses after perfusion of the spinal cord [16]. An important aspect of these findings was that the inhibition is selective for nociceptive information and that the effect is not antagonized by naloxone. This latter finding is particularly significant for clinical use because it suggests that somatostatin will be effective in the face of opiate tolerance.

Chrubasik et al. [2] were the first to test somatostatin for its antinociceptive effects in humans. They found that when given as a bolus or by continuous intrathecal infusion, it markedly reduced pain experienced by cancer patients. This reduction was in the face of opiate tolerance and was not reversed by naloxone. Chrubasik has expanded his investigations to include more patients as well as patients experiencing postoperative pain and found similar results [1]. The use of native somatostatin is limited by a number of practical considerations. It is an unstable compound, so long-term use in a drug pump is not possible. Furthermore, it is rapidly degraded by enzymes in the spinal cord, so relatively high concentrations are necessary. The compound is also expensive and little is available for general medical use. Finally, some studies suggest that at large doses it will be neurotoxic [6, 10], although Chrubasik [1] showed that at the dosage needed clinically it does not cause neurotoxicity.

The solution to these problems is to use octreotide (Sandostatin, Sandoz Pharmaceuticals), a somatostatin analogue that is commercially available for systemic use for endocrine disease. It was specifically designed to not be enzymatically degraded so its effects would be more long-lasting [14]. We tested it in an implanted drug pump at 37° C (SynchroMed, Model 8611, Medtronic, Inc.) and found it to be stable [13]. Chronic intrathecal and intraventricular infusions were performed in rats, dogs, and primates, and octreotide was not neurotoxic at rates up to 40 μg/h. On the basis of this information we received permission from the Food and Drug Administration to perform human investigations.

The goal of the initial clinical studies was to see if chronic intrathecal octreotide had any effect on human nociception. We studied cancer patients who were already receiving intrathecal morphine or were planning to receive such treatment; our patients were already on large systemic and/or intrathecal doses of opiates and still having pain. Thus switching them to intrathecal octreotide also allowed us to make a judgement as to whether the drug works in the face of opiate tolerance.

Details on the implantation, technique, screening criteria, and outcome measures in cancer patients are provided in previous publications [12]. Patients were informed about the new drug trial and were treated in a non-blinded prospective manner. The abbreviated case histories of six patients are as follows.

Case 1

A 65-year-old woman with colon cancer had throbbing pain in her leg and burning and tingling in her rectum and low back and leg due to recurrent tumor. Oral morphine caused significant difficulty in voiding as well as drowsiness. She was the first patient to be tried on intrathecal octreotide. The oral narcotics, intrathecal dosages of octreotide and the visual analog pain scores are shown in Fig. 1 (left) for the 13-day trial period. Good pain relief was achieved at 5 μg/h but was even better at 10 μg/h. She had no side effects, and as the oral narcotics were eliminated she was able to void normally.

Case 2

A squamous cell carcinoma of the gluteus area was causing a severe throbbing pain in the buttock and leg in a 36-year-old man. Ibuprofen, corticosteroids and increasing doses of oral morphine did not provide adequate pain relief. The patient's response to intrathecal octreotide is shown in Fig. 1 (middle). At the time of discharge from the hospital he was receiving 20 μg/h and could reduce his oral narcotics ten-fold and had better pain control. His activities of daily living dramatically increased because he could walk better and sit for longer periods. He died 33 days later due to septic shock, having had adequate pain control.

Case 3

A 54-year-old man with small-cell cancer of the lung had left chest pain; in an effort to treat this an intercostal block had resulted in a constant tingling

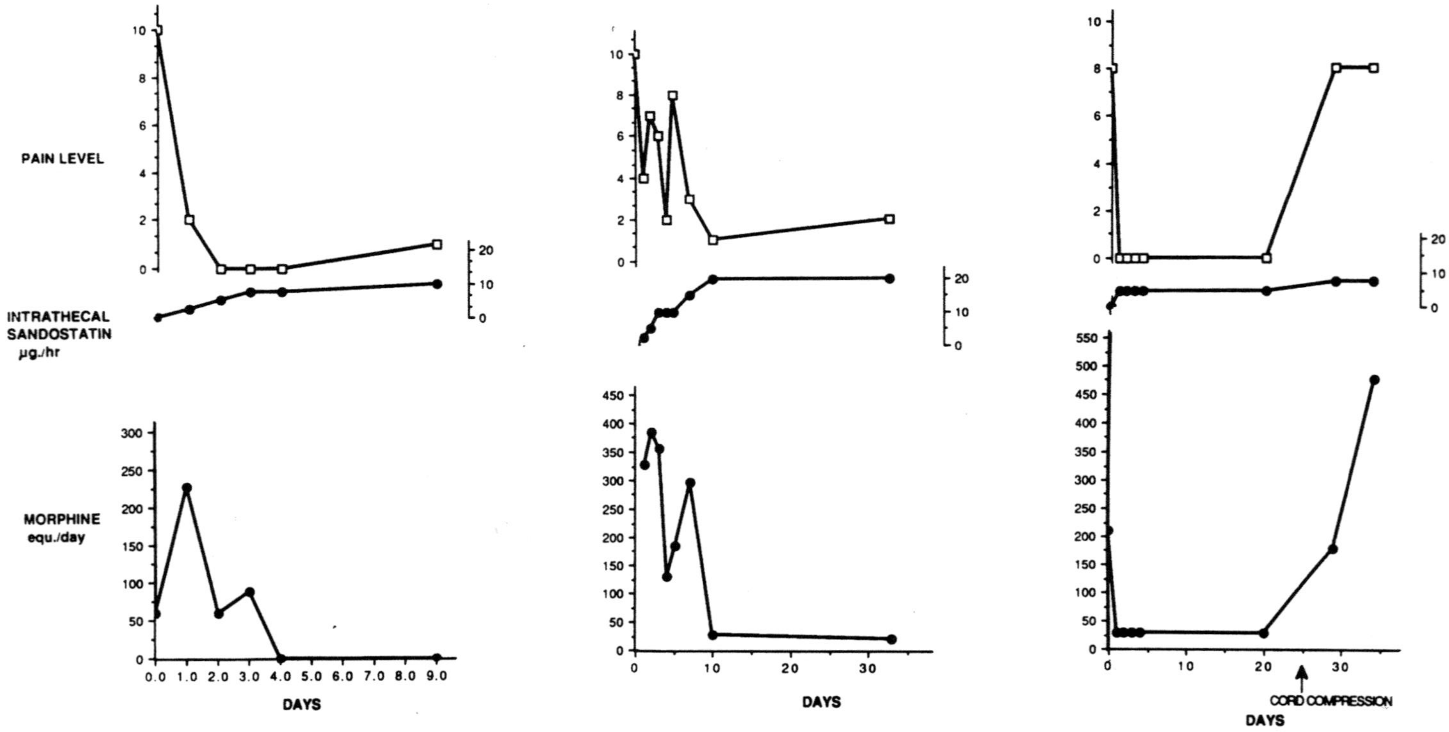

Fig. 1. Patients treated with intrathecal octreotide. Pain level is the visual analog scale rating. Octreotide infusion is in µg/h. Morphine is oral equivalent doses of milligrams of morphine/day. Case 1 *(left)*, Case 2 *(middle)*, Case 3 *(right)*

sensation in his left arm. Intrathecal octreotide at 5 μg/h relieved the somatic chest pain and he was able to reduce oral narcotics by a factor of 7 (Fig. 1, right). However, his left arm tingling became a major discomfort. After a month his pain recurred when a spinal metastasis caused a complete block at T2. Intrathecal medications had to be replaced with high oral doses which were not satisfactory. This case suggests that neurogenic tingling pain is not responsive to octreotide. Also the drug has to reach the spinal level of pain to work; once a block occurred, the pain recurred.

Case 4

A 61-year-old man had colon cancer and invasion of tumor into the retropelvic region. His perirectal and scrotal pain was poorly relieved by 240 mg/day oral morphine and this dose caused lethargy and confusion. He had good relief of pain with intrathecal morphine for 1 year but then developed tolerance, escalating rapidly from 7–12 mg/day to 36 mg/day without adequate relief. Octreotide was given instead of intrathecal morphine and his pain improved (Fig. 2, left). One month later he had an emergency laparotomy for a bowel obstruction during which the catheter from the drug pump kinked stopping delivery of the drug.

This case demonstrates that octreotide can work in spite of clear morphine tolerance. The 36 mg/day intrathecal morphine was replaced by 10 μg/day of octreotide, and at the same time oral narcotics could also be significantly lowered.

Case 5

A 61-year-old man suffered from abdominal and low back pain due to metastatic colorectal cancer. At 1200 mg/day oral morphine he experienced constipation and extreme lethargy. He was given intrathecal octreotide for a total of 76 days (Fig. 2, middle). Through most of this treatment period he had good pain control but toward the end, as his disease progressed, the octreotide and oral morphine had to be increased. When he no longer could swallow, continuous subcutaneous morphine had to be given. It seems that in this patient, as in other cancer patients we have treated, intrathecal medications may not provide enough relief for the generalized discomfort which occurs terminally.

Case 6

A 67-year-old man with metastatic colon cancer dveloped leg and buttock pain; a large presacral mass eroding into the sacrum was found on CT

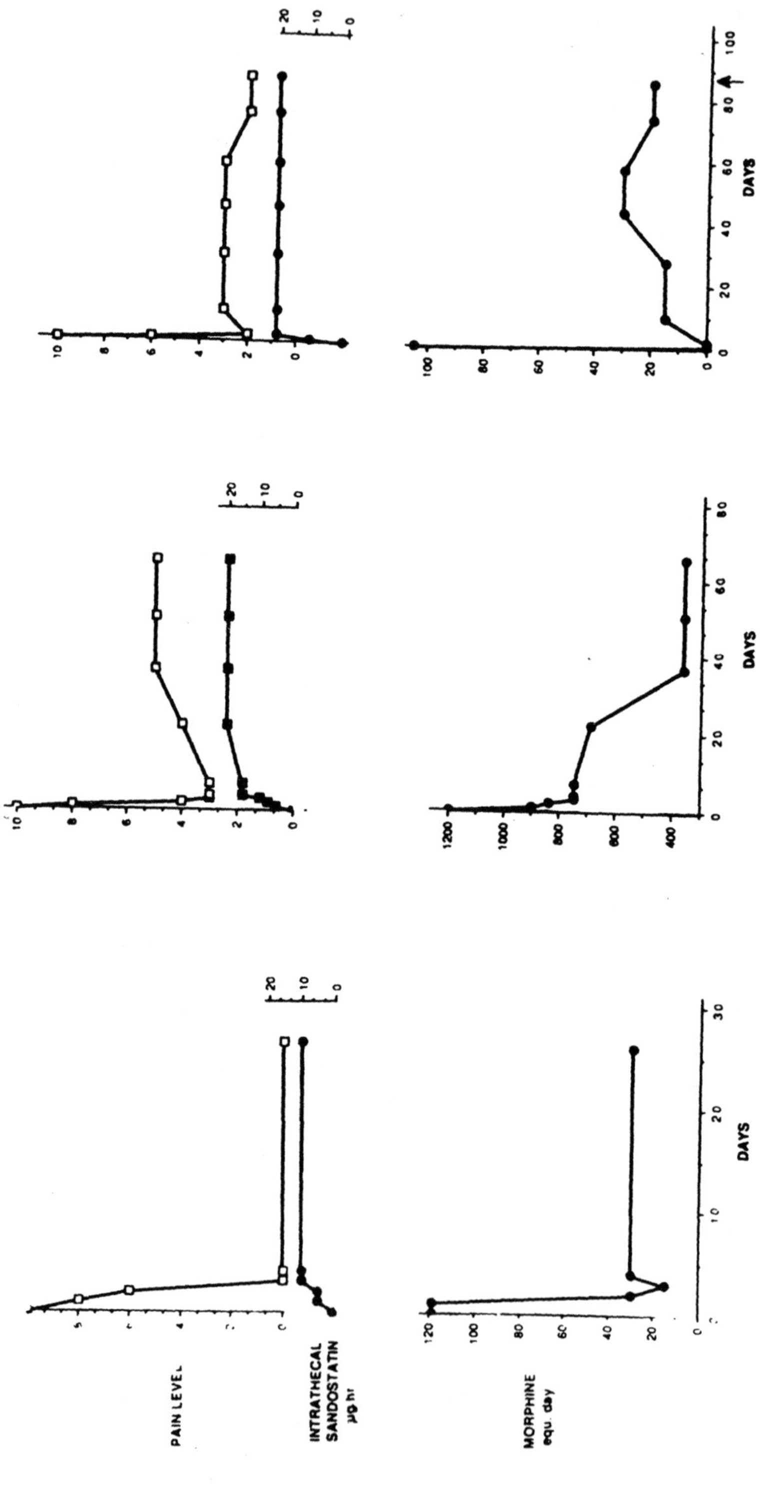

Fig. 2. As Fig. 1. Case 4 *(left)*, Case 5 *(middle)*, Case 6 *(right)*

scanning. Oral narcotics caused drowsiness and urinary retention. Intrathecal octreotide at 20 μg/h allowed him to decrease his oral morphine seven fold and afforded him good pain relief (Fig. 2, right). At 44 days cord compression developed, but with steroids his pain was relieved. When the steroids were later stopped the pain increased rapidly again.

These six cases strongly suggest that octreotide, if given intrathecally at rates from 5 to 20 μg/h, provides good relief of cancer pain. Furthermore, such results may be achieved in the face of opiate tolerance. This experience is not enough to conclude anything more than that the drug seems promising and that further trials are necessary. More prospective studies need to be performed at other centers, and if successful, a blinded comparison to intrathecal morphine could be done.

The importance of these observations is that they demonstrate how potent intrathecal delivery of medication can be in effecting spinal cord mediated pain. Figure 3 is a diagram showing the wide variety of inhibitory and excitatory interneurons which effect dorsal horn neurotransmission. A number of these pathways have already been investigated pharmacologically (using opiates, clonidine, and baclofen). Some of these drugs have significant side effects, such as hypotension caused by clonidine [4]. Others (like baclofen) which theoretically should work, do not produce pain relief [11]. Clearly many appropriate peptides or their agonists or antagonists exist and remain to be tested. However, before such testing is done in humans, animal studies are necessary. Long-term intrathecal infusion of peptides can cause neurotoxic damage, especially because of the high concentrations which are achieved. Only after high infusion rates over several months have proven to be safe in animal experiments should patients be given the medication. When human trials are performed, bolus administration should be avoided because of drug transport in the CSF up the neuraxis and local toxicity from acute, extemely high concentrations. The assumption should not be made that bolus administration will give an accurate idea of the effects of chronic infusion. With these reservations in mind, our preliminary finding with octreotide for cancer pain should encourage further investigations of peptides, which can modify nociception in the spinal cord.

Note. Much of this material will appear as a report in *Pain.* The preclinical animal trials are detailed in that article and the cases are the same.

These studies could not have been performed without the participation of Judith A. Paice, R.N., M.S., and Jeffrey S. Kroin, Ph.D., at Chicago's Rush-Presbyterian-St. Luke's Medical Center. We thank Sandoz and especially Dr. Richard Elton for providing octreotide, and Medtronic, Inc., for technical help with implanted pumps.

The author does not have a financial interest in either the drug or the pump technology. Permission for these studies was granted by the Food and Drug Administration and the Rush H.I.C. Patients gave informed consent.

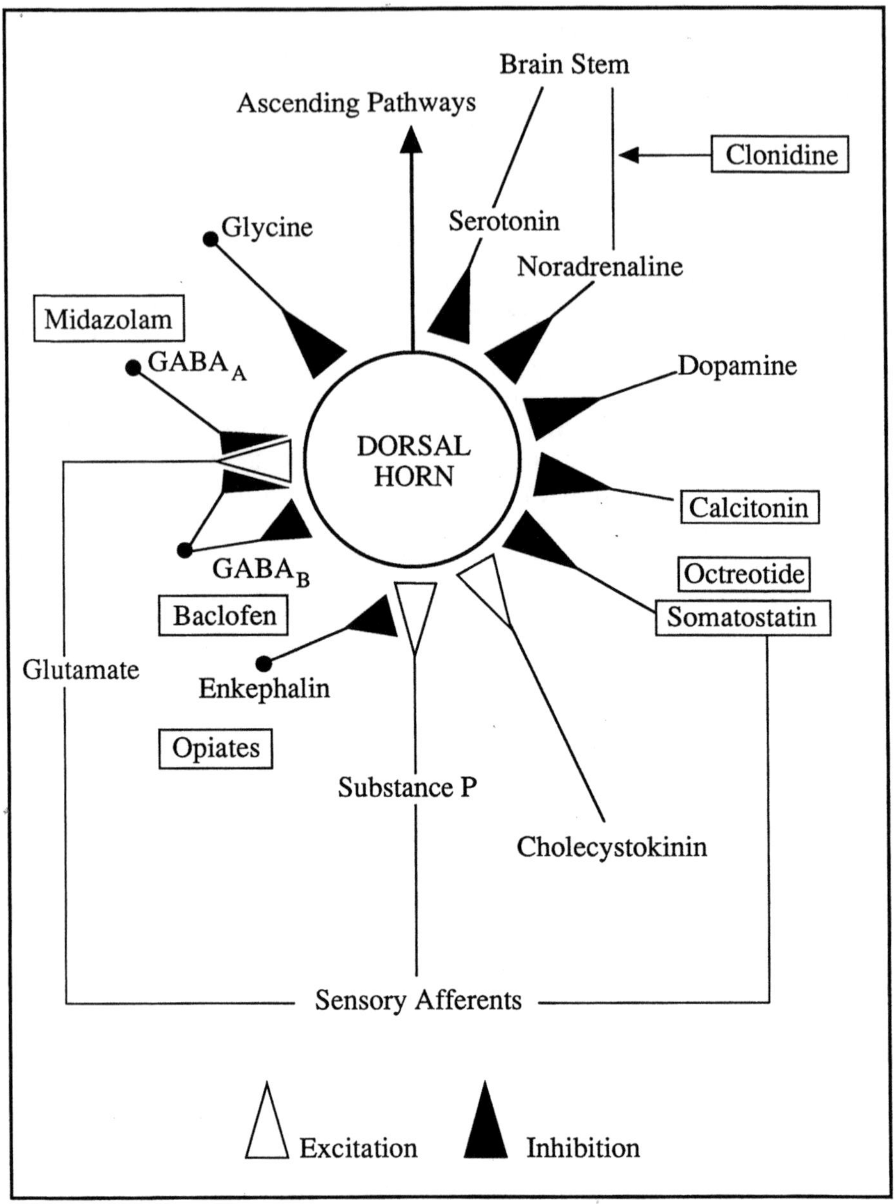

Fig. 3. The multiple interneural pathways that lead to dorsal horn neurons and that might potentially influence nociception

References

1. Chrubasik J (1985) Spinal infusion of opiates and somatostatin. Hygieneplan, Oberursel, FRG

2. Chrubasik J, Meynadier J, Blond S et al (1984) Somatostatin, a potent analgesic. Lancet 2:1208–1209
3. Coombs DW, Fratkin JD, Meier FA (1985) Neuropathologic lesions and CSF morphine concentrations during chronic continuous intraspinal morphine infusion. A clinical and post-mortem study. Pain 22:337–351
4. Coombs DW, Sanders RL, Lachance D et al. (1985) Intrathecal morphine tolerance: use of intrathecal clonidine, DADLE, and intraventricular morphine. Anesthesiology 62:358–363
5. Dahm LS, Beric A, Dimitrijevic MR et al (1989) Direct spinal effect of a benzodiazepine (midazolam) on spasticity in man. Stereotact Funct Neurosurg 53:85–94
6. Gaumann DM, Yaksh TL (1988) Intrathecal somatostatin in rats: antinociception only in the presence of toxic effects. Anesthesiology 68:733–742
7. Griffiths EC, Jeffcoate SL, Holland DL (1977) Inactivation of somatostatin by peptidases in different areas of the rat brain. Actra Endocrinol (Copenh) 85:1–10
8. Kroin JS (1988) Which drugs, what space? Ann NY Acad Sci 531:40–47
9. Krukoff TL, Ciriello J, Calaresu FR (1986) Somatostatin-like immunoreactivity in neurons, nerve terminals, and fibers of the cat spinal cord. J Comp Neurol 243:13–22
10. Long JB (1988) Spinal subarachnoid injection of somatostatin causes neurological deficits and neuronal injury in rats. Eur J Pharmacol 149:287–296
11. Penn RD (1992) Intrathecal baclofen for spasticity of spinal origin: seven years' experience. J Neurosurg (in press)
12. Penn RD, Paice JA, Gottshalk W et al (1984) Cancer pain relief using chronic morphine infusion: early experience with a programmable implanted drug pump. J Neurosurg 61:302–306
13. Penn RD, Paice JA, Kroin JS (1992) Octreotide: a potent new non-opiate analgesic for intrathecal infusion. Pain (in press)
14. Pless J, Bauer W, Briner W et al (1986) Chemistry and pharmacology of SMS 201–995, a long-acting octapeptide analogue of somatostatin. Scand J Gastroenterol Suppl 21:54–64
15. Randic M, Miletic V (1978) Depressant actions of methionine-enkephalin and somatostatin in the cat dorsal horn neurones activated by noxious stimuli. Brain Res 152:196–202
16. Sandkühler J, Fu Q-G, Helmchen C (1990) Spinal somatostatin superfusion in vivo affects activity of cat nociceptive dorsal horn neurons: comparison with spinal morphine. Neuroscience 34:565–576

Biostimulation Techniques for Cancer Pain Management

Winston C. V. Parris

Cancer pain, unlike chronic benign pain, is almost always associated with a specific pathological lesion. That lesion may result from tumor invasion, pressure on a viscus, infiltration of vessels, bony involvement, surgical scarring, or the effects of radiotherapy. Like chronic benign pain, cancer pain may be associated with behavioral aberrations that may cloud the perception of the actual pain, occasionally resulting in amplification of perceived pain. Superimposed on those behavioral features of chronic cancer pain are some intrinsic features which may further augment the patient's perception of pain. Those features include despair, doom, and death issues. Like chronic benign pain, the most effective approach for dealing with chronic cancer pain is to utilize a multidisciplinary approach.

Cancer pain may be the result of a pathological process that is usually progressive or that may produce irreversible and unacceptable pathophysiological changes. As a consequence, the therapeutic interventions utilized to control cancer pain are usually more aggressive and invasive than may be in patients with chronic benign pain. Some of these modalities include radical surgery, innovative medical therapies, aggressive use of narcotic analgesics, or the use of neurolytic procedures. In recent times, renewed interest in the application of biostimulation techniques has demonstrated that these techniques per se may be effective in a large number of cases and furthermore that the complications of biostimulation techniques are usually negligible.

A variety of biostimulation techniques are available for treating patients with chronic cancer pain. Further, the cost/benefit ratio of these techniques makes them attractive modalities. These biostimulation techniques include:

1. Transcutaneous electrical nerve stimulation (TENS)
2. Peripheral nerve stimulation
3. Acupuncture
4. Acupressure
5. Auriculotherapy
6. Physical therapy
7. Movement therapy
8. Vibration therapy
9. Magnetic field therapy

10. Low power laser modulation
11. Laser-TENS therapy
12. Ultrasonic techniques
13. Dorsal column stimulation
14. Deep brain stimulation
15. Heat therapy
16. Ice massage
17. Ancient methods

One of the appealing aspects of these modalities is their relative absence of major complications and the fact that, when effective in a particular patient, the results can be dramatic.

Before considering the different biostimulation modalities individually, some general comments and principles should be considered regarding these techniques. The biostimulation techniques in modern pain medicine today have historic antecedents in that a version of biostimulation was used from as far back as the Socratic era. Electrical stimulation, generated by the electric torpedo fish *(Scribonius longus),* was first reported to be used in patients who had arthritis and headache. The subsequent development of leyden jar condensers and electrostatic generators resulted in the reintroduction of electrotherapy in the late Middle Ages [1]. Since that period, electric therapy has been largely ignored and used mainly by charlatans.

The publication of the classic work on the gate control theory by Melzack and Wall [2] in 1965 rejuvenated biostimulation and in fact, provided a scientific basis for explaining the mechanisms and efficacy of biostimulation techniques for pain management. The gate control therapy focused attention on the important role of the dorsal horn of the spinal cord in modulating sensory transmission. This theory postulates that pain is transmitted to the spinal cord via the small unmyelinated primary afferent fibers (C fibers) and may be inhibited by electrical activity generated via large myelinated primary afferent fibers (A fibers). The inhibitory effect of the A afferent fiber input on C fiber evoked activity has been confirmed electrophysiologically, clinically, and behaviorally. It is this fundamental principle that is applied and utilized in most biostimulation techniques. It is important to point out that alternative mechanisms of action may be applicable in other individual techniques.

Various kinds of electrical stimulation are available and this variability is achieved by alterations of the components of the electrical stimulation device. Most electrical stimulation devices consist of a pulse generator, an amplifier, and electrodes. Different intensities of electrical stimulation may be obtained by varying the pulses produced by the pulse generator, the amount of current available for stimulation, and the amount of impedance of the electrodes and the underlying tissues separating in the electrodes from the peripheral nerves. Thus, fundamental changes in electrical stimulation would be determined by current frequency, and pulse width.

One of the prerequisites for successful electrical stimulation for pain relief is the production of nonpainful paresthesia. Nonpainful paresthesia may be produced by the following techniques:

1. Transcutaneous nerve stimulation using surface electrodes applied to different areas of the skin
2. Peripheral nerve stimulation using electrodes implanted directly on a nerve
3. Peripheral nerve stimulation through subcutaneously implanted electrodes
4. Cutaneous application of a vibrator to activate rapidly adapting low threshold afferents
5. Stimulation of the dorsal columns either directly or through the dura via antidromic activation of primary afferent collateral nerves

Typically, an ideal electrical stimulator (TENS) should consist of a device that is portable, robust, and small, but not so small so as to make its use difficult in elderly patients. The power source should be rechargeable batteries, and in the case of implantable devices the stimulator must have a radiofrequency transmitter that can signal to a coil receiver located subcutaneously. The character of the electrodes is also important, since they largely determine the quality of the electrical stimulation transmitted to the applied surface. The impedance of the underlying tissues and skin is very important since it ultimately affects electrode performance and, consequently, the amount of pain relief obtained.

Like other forms of pain therapy, biostimulation techniques may have significant placebo components. Unfortunately, initial studies of TENS and peripheral nerve stimulation did not take these factors into consideration [3]. Thus, those studies have been regarded by many scientists as flawed. However, recent randomized double-blind controlled studies [4] using TENS devices have confirmed the validity of earlier clinical studies. Thus, notwithstanding the significant placebo component, biostimulation techniques (including TENS and peripheral nerve stimulation) have been shown to be effective in controlling chronic pain.

Bourke et al. [5] demonstrated that patients who received TENS preoperatively required reduced concentrations of halothane to maintain satisfactory anesthesia during hand surgery. Thorsteinsson et al. [6] showed that TENS was three times more effective than placebo in treating the pain of chronic neuropathy. Pike [7] in 1978 showed that narcotic requirements of patients postoperatively were significantly decreased if these patients had been treated intraoperatively with TENS. Ali et al. [8] further demonstrated that pulmonary function studies including measurement of postoperative arterial oxygen tension, vital capacity, and functional residual capacity in patients treated with TENS for upper abdominal surgery showed significant depression compared to patients who were sham-stimulated. All these studies demonstrate that biostimulation techniques (especially TENS and peripheral nerve stimulation) are much more effective than placebo in treating chronic pain.

Transcutaneous Electrical Nerve Stimulation

Of all the biostimulation devices available, TENS is the one most widely used, most widely studied, and most popular with patients. All different kinds of stimulation have been used to treat patients, varying from low frequencies (1–5 Hz to 100–150 Hz). However, elegant studies by Mannheimer and Carlsson [9] have demonstrated that a frequency of approximately 70 Hz is very effective for the majority of patients with chronic pain. Melzack [10] has demonstrated that high-intensity, low-frequency stimulation, while effective in managing chronic pain, may produce unpleasant muscle contractions.

A frequent problem that has been observed in most patients treated with TENS is that there appears to be a loss of efficacy with time. That observation varies from patient to patient, but has been documented in several studies. In a 7-year follow-up study, Bates and Nathan [11] demonstrated that TENS was effective in treating a variety of chronic pain patients, but that a gradual decrease in efficacy was observed in approximately 25% of the patients.

With regard to factors predictive of outcome of therapy, Johansson et al. [12] demonstrated that patients with pain in the extremities responded better than patients with axial pain. Further, they also demonstrated that age and sex were not useful as predictors of outcome of therapy. First, the types of pain that were least suitable for treatment with TENS would include axial, diffuse, psychogenic, and central pain states. For patients with chronic cancer pain, it should be emphasized that TENS may be used alone or as an adjunct to other well-documented treatment modalities in an attempt to supplement their efficacy.

The use of TENS is remarkably free from complications and serious side effects. However, there are a few problems that may occur especially following prolonged use of TENS. These include:

1. development of an allergic dermatitis, which may be a reaction to the adhesive tape holding the TENS electrodes in place;
2. mild erythema in the area of stimulation;
3. a burning or pricking sensation under the area covered by the electrode if an insufficient amount of electrolyte gel is used; and
4. an increase in pain during treatment in patients treated with TENS for the pain of brachial plexus avulsion injury.

Fortunately, increasing pain is usually immediately reversed after the discontinuation of TENS stimulation [13].

There are very few absolute contraindications to TENS. The only absolute contraindications is in patients with pacemakers or with other implanted electrical devices that may be affected by the electrical field generated by the stimulator.

Peripheral Nerve Stimulation

Sweet and Wepsic [14] were the first to use implanted peripheral nerve simulators. Picaza et al. [15] demonstrated that 20 out of 23 patients obtained moderate to dramatic pain relief following implanted peripheral nerve simulators. Most of his patients were postspinal surgery patients, but they also included patients with causalgia, syringomyelia, compression neuropathy, and phantom limb pain. The nerves that were usually stimulated included the peroneal, ulnar, sciatic, occipital, obturator, and pudendal nerves.

Early electrodes were the wrap-around cuff electrodes, but those electrodes had a potential problem of compressing the nerve or of movement and consequently there was a high rate of complications that included infection, equipment malfunction, and postoperative tenderness. In an attempt to bypass those potential complications Nashold [16] adopted a new form of electrode. His study showed that button electrodes were not associated with significant complications as were present with the wrap-around cuf electrodes, but that 50% of his patients required additional surgery in order to improve the position of the stimulating electrode. Thus, while peripheral nerve stimulation is effective for some patients with chronic pain, the technical problems associated with this operation and also the potential complications associated with those procedures suggest that the technique should only be reserved for a select group of patients and be performed by a neurosurgical expert.

The mechanism of action of peripheral nerve stimulation is not precisely known. However, current electrophysiological research in animals has demonstrated that segmental cutaneous A fiber stimulation selectively inhibits C fiber and noxious evoked activity in dorsal horn neurons of spinalized animals. Those observations have been confirmed in man where it has been demonstrated that A fiber stimulation reduces noxious stimulation. In other words, stimulation reduces A δ-evoked flexion reflexes in man. Chan and Tsang [17] have demonstrated that stimulation of myelinated primary afferent A fibers modifies the response of the spinal cord to noxious stimuli and that the analgesic effect of this stimulation is far superior to that of placebo stimulation. The precise mechanism by which A fiber input activates local inhibitory circuits within the spinal cord is not known. Woolf and Wall [18] have suggested that primary afferent stimulation produces depolarization, resulting in the release of a presynaptic inhibitory transmitter which ultimately diminishes the terminal synaptic effectiveness. It is also speculated that the A fiber stimulation produces an excitatory postsynaptic potential and an inhibitory postsynaptic potential complex in several dorsal horn neurons. Further, it is possible that there may be several interneurons that may be responsible for producing the pre- and postsynaptic inhibitions.

Another possible mechanism of action of peripheral nerve stimulation in controlling pain is the possibility that A fiber stimulation may activate some descending inhibitory pathways from the brainstem. Those descending inhibitory mechanisms may contribute further to extrasegmental stimulation-produced analgesia. Other possible mechanisms of action include the role of endogenous opioids in primary afferent mediated inhibitions. The fact that naloxone fails to reverse the analgesic effect of high-frequency TENS and peripheral nerve stimulation in patients with both acute and chronic pain suggests that opioid receptors may not be involved in the analgesia resulting from peripheral nerve stimulation. Thus, although the precise role of opioid mechanisms are unknown, it is likely that nonopioid mechanisms may be involved. The inhibitory transmitter γ-aminobutyric acid (GABA) has been implicated, though not positively identified, as playing a role in the mechanism of action of peripheral nerve stimulation.

In clinical practice it has been demonstrated that the fibers activated by TENS and peripheral nerve stimulation are most exclusively A delta afferents. Further, other studies have shown that A α stimulation produces uncomfortable high-intensity stimulation, while the stimulation of A β afferents is more tolerable. It is not precisely clear whether the stimulation produced by A β and A δ afferents have corresponding inhibitory effects at the spinal cord level. Those inhibitory mechanisms operate on the spinothalamic tract cells and the flexion reflex pathways. In addition to the analgesic effect of the inhibition of those reflexes, there are two other peripheral effects that may occur as a result of peripheral nerve stimulation. These include the diminished sensitizing action that noradrenaline may have on injured axons and on axon terminals in inflamed tissue by interrupting the reflex sympathetic circuit. Another possible effect is that there could be an increase in blood flow secondary to peripheral stimulation, producing an increase in wound healing. Thus, it is clear that peripheral nerve stimulation not only affects the somatosensory pathways but, also, may affect the autonomic nervous system.

Acupuncture

Acupuncture is an ancient form of Chinese medicine that has been practiced for over 2000 years. It involves the insertion of fine needles (gold, silver, and steel) into specific points along the skin. The needles may be twirled or stimulated electrically and the resulting effect is the production of analgesia. The fundamental theory of acupuncture [19] analgesia is built on the principle that different diseases and various pain syndromes are the result of discord between Yin (spirit) and Yan (blood) that flow along certain predetermined areas called channels or "meridians". It has been determined that there are approximately 361 points that lie on 14 meridians in the body. Most of these points correspond to various internal organs and sensation or stimuli relating to these organs can be effected at those points.

Acupuncture was first introduced to the Western world by the Dutch physician, Willem Ten Rhyne, in 1683. Around 1972, after President Nixon visited the People's Republic of China, a renewed interest in acupuncture occurred in the USA and Europe. It was particularly exciting to explore the use of acupuncture analgesia for surgery. A great deal of that interest was dissipated after it was determined that acupuncture was not an effective substitute for anesthesia. In China, approximately 5–10% of surgeries are performed on selected patients using acupuncture. However, acupuncture has been shown to be effective in managing various pain syndromes notably low back pain, neuralgias, and myofascial pain. It has recently been demonstrated by Nathan [20] that nerves rather than meridians are essential for effective pain relief by acupuncture.- The importance of afferent transmission to achieve analgesia was demonstrated by the fact that local anesthetic infiltration of selected acupuncture points blocks the analgesic effect that could be obtained by acupuncture. Reichmanis and Becker [21] demonstrated that the acupuncture effect on pain is significantly greater than that of placebo stimulation. Since then, several studies have corroborated this observation.

It has also been demonstrated that this effect need not necessarily be produced by acupuncture needles alone, but that intense electric stimulation, heat, and a variety of other intense sensory inputs can achieve the same effect. In fact, that has been the putative basis for *acupressure, vibration therapy, heat therapy, ice massage, auriculotherapy, laser therapy, and ultrasound therapy*. The concept is categorized as *hyperstimulation analgesia*. Intense TENS can produce lasting analgesia in which the duration of pain relief outlasts the period of stimulation by several hours and occasionally, days or even months. The utilization of hyperstimulation analgesia in the management of myofascial pain syndrome has been so effective that Travell and Rinzler [22] have proposed that trigger points, as reported in the Western medical literature, and corresponding Chinese acupuncture points may be identical. Several clinicians have observed that the effects of nerve blocks may be achieved purely by inserting the needle into specific points and not associated with the injection of local anesthetics. That effect has been called by Lewit [23] the "needle effect". That needle effect has been documented by Travell and others, and in double-blinded controlled studies Frost et al. [24] demonstrated that patients with trigger points in myofascial pain received more pain relief when injected with normal saline than with mepivacaine.

Auriculotherapy

The principle of auriculotherapy has been proposed by the French physican Nogier [25], who postulated that electrical stimulation at points around the outer ear abolishes pain. Several other physicians found that auriculotherapy is effective, whereas Melzack and Katz [26] did not find (in double-blind studies) that auriculotherapy was an effective means of providing pain control. However, they did find that stimulation of certain points in the region of the outer ear produced a sensation of warmth and glowing feelings. Those referred sensations indicate that there were inputs from the outer ear that project into the central integrating instructors that may play a significant role in those sensations. It is possible that those sensations together with strong placebo suggestion may be the basis for the efficacy of auriculotherapy.

The physiological basis for acupuncture and hyperstimulation analgesia may include the following:

1. Moderate to intense sensory input may be applied to the body to alleviate pain.
2. Sensory input is sometimes applied at a slight distance from the site of the pain.
3. Sensory input that is usually of a brief duration may relieve the chronic pain for several days, weeks, or even months.

There are several other biostimulation techniques that may be used in the management of chronic cancer pain. Whereas most of those techniques may operate on the principles described above, it is likely that some techniques may have alternative mechanisms of action. For example, *magnetic field therapy* is proposed to be effective by increasing mitochondrial ATP. It is also possible that the relationship between oxygen free radicals and paramagnetic oxygen in the tissues may be altered by the magnetic field in some unknown way, resulting in analgesia. *Low-power laser modulation* may also have another unique role to play, although its mechanism of action has not been precisely elucidated.

References

1. Kane K, Taub A (1975) A history of local electrical analgesia. Pain 1:125–138
2. Melzack R, Wall PD (1965) Pain mechanisms: a new theory. Science 150:971–979
3. Vander Ark GD, McGrath KA (1975) Transcutaneous electrical stimulation in treatment of postoperative pain. Am J Surg 130:338–340
4. Harrison RF, Woods T, Shore M, Mathews G, Unwin A (1986) Pain relief in labour using transcutaneous electrical nerve stimulation (TENS). A TENS/TENS placebo controlled study in two parity groups. Br J Obstet Gynaecol 93:739–746
5. Bourke DL, Smith BAC, Erickson J, Gwartz B, Lessard L (1984) TENS reduces halothane requirement during hand surgery. Anesthesiology 61:769–772
6. Thorsteinsson G, Stonnington HH, Stillwell GK, Elveback LR (1977) Transcutaneous electrical stimulation: a double-blind trial of its efficacy for pain. Arch Phys Med Rehabil 58:8–13
7. Pike PM (1978) Transcutaneous electrical stimulation: its use in management of postoperative pain. Anaesthesia 33:165–171
8. Ali JA, Yaffee CS, Serretti C (1981) The effect of transcutaneous electric nerve stimulation on postoperative pain and pulmonary function. Surgery 89:507–512
9. Mannheimer C, Carlsson CA (1979) The analgesic effect of transcutaneous electrical nerve stimulation in patients with rheumatoid arthritis. A comparative study of different pulse patterns. Pain 6:329–334

10. Melzack R (1975) Prolonged relief of pain by brief transcutaneous somatic stimulation. Pain 1:357–373
11. Bates JAV, Nathan PW (1980) Transcutaneous electrical nerve stimulation for chronic pain. Anaesthesia 35:817–822
12. Johansson F, Almay BGL, von Knorring L, Terenius L (1980) Transcutaneous electrical nerve stimulation in patients with chronic pain. Pain 9:55–61
13. Wynn Parry CB (1980) Pain in avulsion lesions of the brachial plexus. Pain 9:41–53
14. Sweet WH, Wepsic JG (1968) Treatment of chronic pain by stimulation of fibres of primary afferent neurons. Trans Am Neurol Assoc 93:103–105
15. Picaza JA, Cannon BW, Hunger SE, Boyd AS, Gum J, Maurer D (1975) Pain suppression by peripheral nerve stimulation. I. Observations with transcutaneous stimuli. Surg Neurol 4:105–114
16. Nashold BS (1980) Peripheral nerve stimulation for pain. J Neurosurg 53:132–133
17. Chan CWY, Tsang H (1987) Inhibition of the human flexion reflex by low intensity high frequency transcutaneous electrical nerve stimulation (TENS) has a gradual onset and offset. Pain 28:239–254
18. Woolf CJ, Wall PD (1982) Chronic peripheral nerve section diminishes the primary afferent A-fibre mediated inhibition of rat dorsal horn neurones. Brain Res 242:77–85
19. Kao FF (1973) Acupuncture therapeutics. Eastern, New Haven
20. Nathan PW (1978) Acupuncture analgesia. Trends Neurosci 1:21–23
21. Reichmanis M, Becker RO (1977) Relief of experimentally induced pain by stimulation at acupuncture loci. Comp Med East West 5:281–288
22. Travell J, Rinzler SH (1952) The myofascial genesis of pain. Postgrad Med 11:425–434
23. Lewit K (1979) The needle effect in the relief of myofascial pain. Pain 6:83–90
24. Frost FA, Jessen B, Siggaard-Andersen J (1980) A control, double-blind comparison of mepivacaine injection versus saline injection for myofascial pain. Lancet 1:499–501
25. Nogier PFM (1972) Treatise of auriculotherapy. Maisonneuve, Metz
26. Melzack R, Katz J (1984) Auriculotherapy fails to relieve chronic pain. JAMA 251:1041–1043

GPSR Compliance

The European Union's (EU) General Product Safety Regulation (GPSR) is a set of rules that requires consumer products to be safe and our obligations to ensure this.

If you have any concerns about our products, you can contact us on ProductSafety@springernature.com

In case Publisher is established outside the EU, the EU authorized representative is:

Springer Nature Customer Service Center GmbH
Europaplatz 3
69115 Heidelberg, Germany

Batch number: 10704713

Printed by Printforce, the Netherlands